For years, cardiologist Arthur Agatston urged his patients to lose weight for the sake of their hearts, but every diet was too hard to follow or its restrictions were too harsh. Some were downright dangerous. Nobody seemed to be able to stick with low-fat regimens for any length of time. And a diet is useless if you can't stick with it.

So Dr Agatston developed his own and news of his patients' dramatic successes soon spread far and beyond the confines of his practice. Strangers started calling to ask for a copy of the diet, and local news began featuring stories of its popularity. Soon, the South Beach Diet was a bona fide craze in Miami. And no wonder: South Beach dieters lose 8 to 13 pounds in the first two weeks without feeling hungry, and there's no mandatory exercise. Dr Agatston's simple plan allows you to eat the foods you love – meat and fish, cheese, healthy oils and nuts, vegetables, the right carbohydrates and even sweets. Best of all, you lose weight from your waistline first! It couldn't be easier.

Born in New York in 1947, Arthur Agatston graduated from the University of Wisconsin and trained in various hospitals in the New York area. He moved to Florida in 1979 to join the Mount Sinai Medical Center as Director, Non-invasive Cardiac Laboratory and Director of Cardiac Rehabilitation. He is internationally renowned for his knowledge of heart disease and has developed Electron Beam Technology (EBT) and the 'Agatston Score', which is used worldwide to measure calcium deposits in the heart and vascular system. He is married with two children and lives in Miami Beach.

Also by Dr Arthur Agatston

The South Beach Diet: Good Fats/Good Carbs Counter

THE SOUTH BEACH DIET

The Delicious, Doctor-designed Plan
For Fast and Healthy Weight Loss

Dr A. Agatston

headline

First published in Great Britain in 2003
by HEADLINE BOOK PUBLISHING

Published by arrangement with Rodale, Inc., Emmaus, PA, USA

30 29 28

ISBN 0 7553 1129 9

Typeset in Gill Sans by
Letterpart Limited, Reigate, Surrey

Printed and bound in Great Britain by
Clays Ltd, St Ives plc

Every effort has been made to fulfil requirements
with regard to reproducing copyright material.
The author and publisher will be glad to rectify
any omissions at the earliest opportunity.

HEADLINE BOOK PUBLISHING
A division of Hodder Headline
338 Euston Road
LONDON NW1 3BH

www.headline.co.uk
www.hodderheadline.com

For my wife Sari.
For her support, enthusiasm and love.

contents

acknowledgements

Writing these acknowledgements is frustrating because it is impossible to mention all those who have supported me and influenced my work. But the research that led to the South Beach Diet was a cooperative effort, and I want to recognize those who directly helped. My prevention research began with coronary artery calcium detection through Electron Beam Tomography (EBT). Dr Warren Janowitz was and is a brilliant and essential partner in this project. David King and Dr Manuel Viamonte Jr gave Warren and me great support and advice throughout. When I decided to work with a diet that defied the conventional wisdom, I went first to Marie Almon, a dietitian, who became an invaluable associate. I received great support and counsel from my colleagues and collaborators Drs Gervasio Lamas, Eric Lieberman, Charlie Hennekens, Robert Superko, and Wade Aude.

Kristi Krueger and Jana Ross from WPLG Channel 10 became wonderful partners in bringing the South Beach Diet to the South Florida public. Finally, when the book project was in doubt, along came author, lecturer, and friend Linda Richman, who connected me with my superb agent, Richard Pine.

Thanks also to the various chefs who allowed their creations to be included in this book; these recipes are marked with an asterisk and credited on page 270.

Arthur Agatston

part I

Understanding the South Beach Diet

losing weight, gaining life

The South Beach Diet is not low carb. Nor is it low fat.

The South Beach Diet teaches you to rely on the right carbs and the right fats – the *good* ones – and enables you to live quite happily without the bad carbs and bad fats. As a result, you're going to get healthy and lose weight – somewhere between 8 and 13 pounds in the next two weeks alone.

Here's how you'll do it.

You'll eat normal-size helpings of meat, chicken, turkey, fish, and shellfish.

You'll have plenty of vegetables. Eggs. Cheese. Nuts.

You'll have salads with real olive oil in the dressing.

You'll have three balanced meals a day, and it will be your job to eat so that your hunger is satisfied. Nothing undermines a weight-loss plan more than the distressing sensation that you need more food. No sane eating programme expects you to go through life feeling discomfort. You'll be urged to have snacks in the mid-morning and mid-afternoon, whether you need to or not. You'll have dessert after dinner.

You'll drink water, of course, plus coffee or tea if you wish.

For the next 14 days you *won't* be having any bread, rice, potatoes, pasta, or baked goods. No fruit, even. Before you panic: You'll begin adding those things back into your diet again in two weeks. But for right now, they're off-limits.

No sweets, cake, biscuits, ice-cream, or sugar for two weeks, either. No beer or alcohol of any kind. After this phase you'll be free to drink wine. It's beneficial for a variety of reasons. Not a drop during the first two weeks, however.

Now, if you're the kind of person who lives for pasta or bread or potatoes, or if you believe that you can't get through a day without feeding your sweet tooth (three or four times), let me tell you something: You're going to be shocked at how painlessly two weeks without these foods will pass. The first day or two may be challenging, but once you weather that you'll be fine. It's not that you'll have to fight your urges – during the first week the cravings will virtually disappear. I say this with such confidence only because it's what so many overweight people who have already succeeded on this programme tell me. The South Beach Diet may be new to you, but it has existed for several years, long enough to have helped hundreds of people lose weight easily and keep it off.

So that's Phase 1, the strictest period.

After two weeks of that, you will be somewhere between 9 and 13 pounds lighter than you are today. Most of that weight will come off your mid-section, so right away you'll notice the difference in your clothes. It will be easier to zip your jeans than it's been for some time. That blazer will close without a bulge.

But this will just be the noticeable difference. You won't be able to see that during those two weeks you'll also have changed yourself internally. You will have corrected the way your body reacts to the very foods that made you overweight. There's a switch inside you that had been turned on. Now, simply by modifying your diet, you'll have turned it off. The physical cravings that ruled your eating habits will be gone, and they'll stay away for as long as you stick with the programme. The weight loss doesn't happen because you're trying to eat less. But you'll be eating fewer of the foods that created those bad old urges, fewer of the foods that caused your body to store excessive fat.

As a result of *that* change, you will continue losing weight after the 14-day period ends, even though by then you will have begun adding some of those banished foods back into your life. You'll still be on a diet, but if it's bread you love, you'll have bread. If it's pasta, you'll reintroduce that. Rice or cereal, too. Potatoes. Fruit will definitely be back.

Chocolate? If it makes you feel good, sure. You will have to pick and choose which of these indulgences you permit yourself. You won't be able to have them all, all the time. You'll learn to enjoy them a little differently than before – maybe a little less enthusiastically. But you will enjoy them again soon.

That's Phase 2.

You'll remain in that phase and continue losing weight until you reach your goal. How long it takes depends on how much you need to lose. In Phase 2 people lose, on average, a pound or two a week. Once you hit your target, you'll switch to an even more liberal version of the programme, which will help you to maintain your ideal weight.

That's Phase 3.

That stage is the one that lasts the rest of your life. When you get to that point, you'll notice that this plan feels less like a diet and more like a way of life – you'll be eating normal foods, after all, in normal-size portions. You can then feel free to forget all about the South Beach Diet, as long as you remember to live by its few basic rules.

As you're losing weight and altering how your body responds to food, a third change will be taking place. This one will significantly alter your blood chemistry, to the long-term benefit of your cardiovascular system. You will improve invisible factors that only cardiologists and heart patients worry about. Thanks to this final change, you will substantially increase your odds of living long and well – meaning, you will maintain your health and vitality as you age.

You may start on the South Beach Diet hoping just to lose weight. If you adopt it and stay with it, you will surely accomplish that much. But you'll also do a lot more for yourself, all of it very good. I'm not exaggerating when I say that this diet can, as a fringe benefit, save your life.

chapter two

good carbs, bad carbs

I'm not a diet doctor.

In fact, my career in medicine has been largely devoted to the science of non-invasive cardiac imaging – the development of technology that produces sophisticated pictures of the heart and the coronary blood vessels. This allows us to identify problems and treat them early, before they cause heart attack or stroke. In CT (computerized tomography) scanning all over the world, I'm proud to say, the measure of coronary calcium is called the Agatston Score, and the protocol for calcium screening is often referred to as the Agatston Method. I maintain an active, full-time cardiology practice, both clinical and research.

So how is it I am also responsible for a weight-loss programme that has become a phenomenon in South Florida – a regime that's helped countless women and men, many of them in their twenties and thirties, young enough to be the grandchildren of my usual cardiology patients – get down to string bikini and Speedo swimming trunks shape?

I have to admit, I wasn't prepared to find myself on the receiving end of so much buzz. I'm now regularly stopped by people who have seen my TV news appearances or read about the diet's success in newspapers and magazines. Given South Beach's worldwide image as a mecca of physical beauty and body consciousness and its role as a chic outpost of the fashion industry, it's an unexpected position to find myself in.

This all started, however, as a serious medical undertaking. Back in the mid-nineties I was but one of many cardiologists who had grown disillusioned with the low-fat, high-carbohydrate diet recommended by the American

Heart Association in order to help us all eat properly and maintain healthy weight. None of the low-fat regimes of that era seemed to work reliably, especially over the long haul. My concern was not with my patients' appearance, of course: I wanted to find a diet that would help prevent or reverse the myriad heart and vascular problems that stem from obesity.

I never found such a diet. Instead, I developed it myself.

Today, I feel nearly as comfortable in the world of nutrition as I do among cardiologists. I speak regularly before physicians, researchers, and other health-care professionals who devote their lives to helping patients eat sensibly and lose weight. Although my interest in diet started from the therapeutic perspective, I see now that the cosmetic benefits of losing weight are extremely important because they so effectively motivate the young *and* the old – even more than the promise of a healthy heart, it often seems. The psychological lift that comes from an improved appearance benefits the entire person, and in turn keeps many a patient from backsliding – which, in the end, benefits cardiovascular health, my only goal when this journey began.

What started as a part-time foray into the world of nutrition has led me to devise a simple, medically sound diet that works, without stress, for a large percentage of those who try it, a programme that has been scientifically studied (as few diets ever are) and proven effective both for losing weight and for getting and keeping a healthy cardiovascular system.

Back when this all began, of course, I had no idea what would ensue. All I knew was that many of my patients – more of them every year – were overweight and that their condition was a big part of their cardiac burden. I could treat them with all the newest medications and procedures, but until they got their diet under control we were often fighting a losing battle. Their eating habits contributed to blood chemistry that was dangerously high in cholesterol and triglycerides, the leading factors in blocked arteries and inflammation of the blood vessels. And there was another, not terribly well-understood diet-related problem that they shared, a silent, so-called *metabolic* syndrome (prediabetes) found in close to half of all Americans who suffer heart attacks.

Searching for the right weight-loss plan

My journey to disease prevention through diet actually began when my education as a cardiologist did, 30 years ago. During my training in the late

1970s, I looked forward to treating patients with heart disease – despite the fact that we didn't have many preventative weapons in our arsenal. I asked the most respected cardiologist I knew this question: 'What is the best way to prevent heart disease?' His answer: 'Pick the right parents.' If you inherited the gene for cardiac longevity, you were likely to live to a ripe old age. If heart disease struck early in your family, there was not much you could do to change your destiny.

Then, in 1984, I attended a course at the Heart House in Bethesda, Maryland, the national headquarters of the American College of Cardiology. There, I heard a lecture by a brilliant researcher and charismatic teacher, Bill Castelli, who headed the world-famous Framingham Heart Study. Dr Castelli told us about the results of the recently completed National Institutes of Health (NIH)-sponsored Lipid Research Clinics Primary Prevention Trial (LRCPPT). This was the very first study to prove that lowering cholesterol via diet could reduce heart attacks. At the time, the only known treatment for high cholesterol was an unpleasant, grainy powder known as a resin, which was taken several times a day before meals. Therefore, we were all very excited when Dr Castelli told the conference that if we put patients on the very first American Heart Association diet, we could lower their cholesterol and end the scourge of heart disease in America.

We physicians all returned home filled with fervour, ready to guide our patients to restored cardiac health and dietary wisdom. I came back to Miami confident in my newfound knowledge of how to save my patients' lives. My wife and I even joked that with heart disease out of the picture, I might be better off switching to a growth specialty, like plastic surgery. It wasn't long before I learned that unemployment as a cardiologist was going to be unlikely.

I began counselling my patients on the low-fat, high-carbohydrate diet advocated by the American Heart Association, but the results fell far below my expectations. Often, there was an initial modest improvement in total cholesterol with mild weight loss. This invariably was followed by a return of cholesterol to its previous level or higher, along with a return of the lost weight. This scenario was not only my experience but also that of my colleagues. It was reflected in the many diet-cholesterol trials documented in the literature that showed our inability to sustain cholesterol and/or weight reductions using low-fat, high-carbohydrate diets. There were no convincing studies showing that the American Heart Association diet saved lives.

Over the years I had suggested most of the highly respected diets out there – going back to Pritikin (see chapter three) and then through the various, more recent, heart-healthy low-fat regimes, including the Ornish plan and several American Heart Association diets – and seen each of them, for different reasons, fail miserably. Either the diets were too difficult to stick with, or the promise of improved blood chemistry and cardiac health remained just that – a promise. Discouraged, I had all but given up on advising my patients about nutrition, because I was unable to suggest anything that actually helped. Like most cardiologists in that period, I turned instead to the statin drugs that were just coming on the market, medications that had proven extremely effective in lowering total cholesterol, if not weight.

But I also decided, as a last-ditch effort, that I would devote some serious study of my own to diet and obesity. Like most physicians, I was not particularly knowledgeable in the science of nutrition. So my first task was to research all the weight-loss programmes out there, the serious scientific ones as well as the trendy attempts that topped the best-seller lists. As I acquired that education, I was also reading in the cardiology literature about the prevalence of something called the insulin resistance syndrome and its effect on obesity and heart health.

The science of success

One side effect of excess weight, we now know, is an impairment of the hormone insulin's ability to do its job of processing fuel, or fats and sugars, properly. This condition is commonly called insulin resistance. As a result, the body stores more fat than it should, especially in the mid-section. We've been genetically conditioned to store fat since the dawn of *homo sapiens*, as a survival strategy to see us through times of famine.

The problem now, of course, is that we never experience the famine end of that equation, only the feast. As a result, we store fat but never require our bodies to burn it off. Much of our excess weight comes from the carbohydrates we eat, especially the highly processed ones found in baked goods, breads, snacks, and other convenient favourites. Modern industrial processing removes the fibre from these foods, and once that's gone their very nature – and how we metabolize them – changes significantly, and for the worse.

Decrease the consumption of those 'bad' carbs, studies showed, and the insulin resistance starts clearing up on its own. Weight begins a fairly rapid decrease, and you begin metabolizing carbs properly. Even the craving for carbs disappears once you cut down on their consumption. Finally, cutting out processed carbs improves blood chemistry, ultimately resulting in lowered triglycerides and cholesterol.

So my eating plan's first principle was to permit good carbohydrates (fruits, vegetables, and whole grains) and curtail the intake of bad carbohydrates (the highly processed ones, for the most part, where all the fibre had been stripped away during manufacturing). We would thereby eliminate a prime cause of obesity. This was in marked contrast to the Atkins Diet, for instance, which bans virtually *all* carbohydrates and leaves the dieter to exist mostly on proteins. That regime also permits limitless saturated fats, the kind found in red meat and butter. These are, as most people know, the bad fats – the ones that can lead to cardiovascular disease, heart attack, and stroke. That hasn't stopped millions of dieters from adopting the plan. But from the moment I learned of it, the diet set off alarm bells in this cardiologist's head. Even if you do lose weight and keep it off, your blood chemistry is bound to suffer from eating so much saturated fat.

My plan cut certain carbohydrates, but not all. In fact, it encouraged eating the good ones. For instance, I banished white flour and white sugar. But our diet permits whole grain breads and cereals and wholemeal pasta. We also prescribe lots of vegetables and fruit. I had a practical reason, beyond their obvious nutritional value and the beneficial fibre they provide, for that decision. Not everyone *wants* to give up vegetables, fruit, bread, and pasta for ever, even in exchange for a regime that allows a pound of bacon for breakfast, followed by a pound of hamburger (with no bun, of course) for lunch, topped by a thick steak for dinner. And if people want bread, pasta, or rice, a humane eating plan should be able to accommodate that desire.

To make up for the overall cut in carbohydrates, my diet permitted ample fats and animal proteins. This decision flew in the face of the famous diets that had been developed specifically for people with heart problems, like Pritikin and Ornish. For a cardiologist, this was skating on thin ice. But my experience with patients showed that those so-called heart-healthy diets were nearly impossible to stick to, because they relied too heavily on the dieters' ability to eat superlow fat over the long haul. The South Beach diet would permit lean beef, pork, veal, and lamb.

The low-fat regime's severe restrictions on meat were unnecessary – the latest studies had showed that lean meat did not have a harmful effect on blood chemistry. Even egg yolks are good for you – they're a source of natural vitamin E and have a neutral-to-favourable effect on our balance between good and bad cholesterol, contrary to what we once believed. Chicken, turkey, and fish (especially the oily ones such as salmon, tuna, and mackerel) were recommended on my diet, along with nuts and low-fat cheeses and yogurt. As a rule, low-fat prepared foods *can* be a bad idea – the fats are replaced with carbs, which are themselves fattening. But dairy products such as cheese, milk, and yogurt that are low fat are exceptions to this rule – they are nutritious and not fattening.

I also allowed plenty of healthy mono- and polyunsaturated fats, like the Mediterranean ones: olive oil, rapeseed oil, and peanut oil. These are the good fats. They can actually reduce the risk of heart attack or stroke. In addition to being beneficial, they taste good and make food palatable. They're filling, too – a major consideration for a diet that promises you won't have to go hungry.

Next, I found a suitable guinea pig for preliminary testing purposes, a middle-aged man who was having trouble keeping his growing paunch under control: me. I went on the diet. I gave up bread, pasta, rice, potatoes. No beer. No fruit even, at least in the very beginning, because it contains high levels of fructose, or fruit sugar. But otherwise I was determined to eat as normally as possible, meaning three meals a day plus snacks when I was hungry.

After just a week, I noticed a difference. I lost almost 8 pounds in those first seven days, and it was easy. I didn't suffer any hunger pangs. No terrible cravings. No noticeable deprivation.

Almost sheepishly, I approached Marie Almon, MSRD, chief clinical dietitian at our hospital, Mount Sinai Medical Center in Miami Beach, and told her of my experiment. She conceded that the low-fat diet we had been recommending to cardiac patients wasn't working. So we took the basic principles I had developed and expanded them into an agreeable eating plan.

Practical solutions

We settled on a few more guidelines, based on my clinical experience and study of the literature. First, we acknowledged the primary failing of diets we had tried with patients: They're too complicated and too rigid. A diet may be medically or nutritionally sound, but if it is hard to live with, if it doesn't take into account how human beings operate – the whole person, not just his or her digestive tract and metabolism – then it is a failure. So this diet would be flexible and simple, with as few rules as possible. It would allow people to eat the way people actually *like* to eat, while improving their blood chemistry and helping them lose weight and maintain the loss over the long run. This means a lifetime, not three months or a year. Only by accomplishing these goals would this pro-gramme make the crucial transition from being a diet to being a lifestyle – a way of living and eating that normal human beings can sustain for the rest of their lives.

With that in mind, we decided that we wouldn't ask people to deny themselves every eating pleasure indefinitely. Typically, once you've gone off track on a diet, once you've strayed, you're on your own – the experts never allow for human frailty or tell you how to accommodate the inevitable slips as part of the plan. As a result, people who cheat a little today usually cheat a little more tomorrow, and then it's a slippery slope down to where the diet's in shambles, you've broken every rule, and you're depressed and discouraged and back at square one. So we make ample use of desserts devised especially by Marie Almon for the programme. These treats are delicious, yet use only 'legal' ingredients.

We also simply recognized that there will be days when you just *need* that chocolate ice-cream or lemon meringue pie. I'm a chocoholic myself, so believe me, I understand. This plan would allow dieters to bend or break the rules, so long as they understand exactly what damage they've done and how to undo it. If the cheating did put a few pounds on, or stall the weight loss, the setback would be minimal and easily repaired, rather than spelling doom. One beauty of the three-phase structure of the South Beach Diet is that you can move easily from one stage to another. If, while in Phase 2, you go on vacation and overindulge in sweets, it's easy to switch back to Phase I for a week, lose the weight those desserts put on, and then return to where you left off in Phase 2.

Finally, people are practical beings. Diets that require complex menus, or supplements taken at certain times of day, or foods eaten in precise combinations, are just too burdensome to sustain for long. Many popular diets are extremely tricky in that regard, despite the fact that there is no basis in science for such complexity. And so they fail. Most of us lead complicated enough lives without having to be within walking distance of a refrigerator every two hours. Nobody wants to carry around a pillbox or a rule book (or both). So this diet would be based on dishes that are easy to make, with ingredients that are commonly found in supermarkets or even most restaurants. The plan requires snacks between meals, but the kind that can be thrown into a briefcase or backpack in the morning and eaten on the run. Our diet is also distinguished by the absence of calorie counts; percentage counts of fats, carbs, and proteins; or even rules about portion size. Our major concern is that dieters eat good carbs and good fats. Once that's all under control, portions and percentages take care of themselves. By choosing the right carbs and the right fats, you simply won't be hungry all the time.

Our diet, we decided, would have to be effective regardless of the dieter's exercise habits. Without a doubt, exercise does increase the body's metabolism, thereby making the diet more efficient. It is also a critical part of any cardiac health plan. However, the South Beach Diet does not depend on exercise in order to work. You'll lose more weight, faster, if you are active on a regular basis. But you'll lose weight even if you're not.

Flexibility and common sense, guided by real science – as opposed to the pop science that often passes for nutrition these days – were the guiding principles of the South Beach Diet. We hoped we had come up with a workable, practical solution to the obesity that plagued so many people we saw in the hospital setting. We believed it would work for most of them. But of course, we wouldn't really know until they tried it.

MY SOUTH BEACH DIET

KAREN G.:

I'VE LOST 2 STONE 2 LB AND KEPT IT OFF.

I had just moved back to Miami Beach from Arizona after getting a divorce. And, of course, everybody in that situation goes on what I call the Divorce Diet – you know, you're going to be dating people for the first time in a long, long time. And those 30 extra pounds you put on during 30 years of marriage? Back when you thought it didn't matter?

Anyway, I read about the South Beach Diet in the newspaper and it sounded easy, so I got all the details. My big thing is that I hate feeling hungry. I just don't like the sensation. In the past, I had been on plenty of low-fat diets, and I *always* felt hungry. On this diet, though, the rule is that if you feel hungry, you eat. When you sit down to a meal, you're supposed to eat until you're satisfied.

Salty and starchy things were always my weakness, much more than sweets – crisps, chips, popcorn. I would go to a supermarket and the first thing I bought was a large bag of popcorn, and by the time I was through shopping it was finished. And I never went to a movie without having buttered popcorn – never, ever, *ever*. I had a husband who wanted dinner from soup to nuts, every night: Salad, meat, potatoes, a vegetable, bread – always bread. For me to sit down in a restaurant and not have bread and butter was a big sacrifice. You know, on most diets they say you can have the bread but not the butter. On this diet you can have the butter, but not the bread. Or if you have the bread, it's whole grain dipped in olive oil instead of slathered with butter.

It wasn't so easy for me in the first few weeks, during the strict phase. I had to cut out all the things I loved – bread, potatoes, rice, pasta, crisps. I actually didn't feel so great. I felt... not bad, exactly, but not completely myself either. For the first three weeks I felt like I was getting all that bad stuff out of my system. And while I never was hungry, I still craved all the things I couldn't have.

I don't even have the desire for them now, though. The cravings went away. Now when I want a salad I can have it – and with dressing on it. *Real* dressing, not some crappy stuff that tastes horrible.

My mother went on the diet when she saw the weight I lost. She's 81 and she's got terrible cholesterol, too. After the first couple of weeks she said, 'You know, I'm feeling hungry.' And I said to her, 'Mom, the point of this diet is that you don't *have* to be hungry. *Eat*. If you're hungry, go get a piece of cheese.' She had assumed that if it's a diet, you're supposed to be hungry. She took my advice and started eating, and she still lost about a stone, which she had never been able to take off before.

I'm pretty born again about this diet. I don't cheat a lot. No pasta at all. No rice at all. I can have brown rice, but I don't like it. No potatoes, except for sweet potatoes, and even then, only baked. And not so often. No sweets. I *have* added bread back, because I still love it. Not every day – maybe two or three times a week. And never white. I'll have wholemeal, or rye, or pumpernickel, but even then I always ask if there's any white flour in it. Because many times, there *is*. Rye bread you buy at the supermarket has white flour in it, for instance. So you have to watch it.

Honestly, the best part about this programme is that there isn't a restaurant I can't go into. For lunch, just about any restaurant can make you a salad with vegetables and cheese or meat or fish in it. You can get chicken salad or tuna salad anywhere, too. I can go to Burger King and get a barbecued chicken sandwich and throw away the bread. I go to an Italian restaurant that fixes me veal parmigiana without the coating – just tomato sauce and cheese on top. We'll go to a steak house and I'll have prawn cocktail and steak with a vegetable – steamed asparagus or green beans, and I can put butter on it, too. I don't overdo it, but it's real butter. And I'll have a salad with blue cheese dressing. And that's not cheating!

I went on the diet three years ago and I've lost 2 stone 2 lb and kept it off. I feel comfortable again. I'm a size 14 now, and I feel fine the way I am. I would love to lose another 10 pounds, but I'm not going to kill myself to do it. I *was* wearing a size 18. So I had to go to the fat-lady store. It's not fun to go to the fat-lady store.

chapter three

a brief history of recent diets

If you're confused about weight-loss programmes, you're not alone. At any given moment, popular diets run the gamut from low fat–high carb to high fat–low carb. Some emphasize high protein. Others require precise combinations of nutrients in each meal. In my medical practice, I've found that a good understanding of the thinking behind a diet leads to high compliance. With that in mind, I'll try to give you a basic grasp of the principles of the South Beach Diet.

First, a brief history, to bring you up to speed.

The modern era of better health through weight loss begins with the American Heart Association diet recommendations that grew out of post-World War II studies done by a pioneering researcher, Dr Ansel Keys of the University of Minnesota. He compared cholesterol and heart attack rates in countries around the world, and found that where there was low intake of fat, people enjoyed better cardiovascular health. This was for the most part true, and it furthered our understanding of how food affects our health.

But it was not entirely true, and it has taken us many years to complete our knowledge of how nutrition and health (especially cardiac health) are connected.

When Dr Keys performed his studies of the relationship between high fat and heart disease, he found an exception on the Greek island of Crete, where there was high intake of fat and yet very low heart attack rates. It ran counter to everything else his studies indicated, and so the Crete exception was ignored. This turned out to be an unfortunate decision.

It was largely on the basis of Dr Keys' findings and other similar studies that national recommendations to lower total fat intake were determined. It was decided at the time not to perform a billion-dollar study that would test the effects of a low-fat diet. Instead, the guidelines were set on the basis of the best evidence available. To be fair, it is difficult to measure the long-term effects of diet on the cardiovascular system. Arteriosclerosis buildup in blood vessel walls takes a lifetime before it is serious enough to cause heart attack or stroke. Thus, the ideal diet study would have taken many years to complete, during which the cost of monitoring study participants could be prohibitive.

There was also a political component to the low-fat guidelines – a kind of 'nutritional correctness' not unlike the political correctness of recent years. The role that a Senate committee chaired by George McGovern played in the writing of our national dietary guidelines was brilliantly documented by journalist Gary Taubes in the journal *Science* in March 2001. The McGovern committee was originally chartered to fight malnutrition, but in the 1970s it switched to a new goal – the prevention of overnutrition. The campaign started with a preconceived notion: Fat was inherently bad, and our overindulgence in it was the major cause of obesity and heart disease in the United States. The committee also tended to suspect that those who did not believe fat was public enemy number one were being unduly influenced by the beef, egg, or dairy industry. The bottom line is that low total fat, high carbohydrate became the orthodoxy, despite the lack of proof that such a diet would improve overall health.

Fats vs carbs: the debate

How has America done since the low-fat, high-carbohydrate diet recommendations? We've got fatter and fatter. In addition, adult-onset diabetes, a sure sign of unhealthy blood chemistry, has become widespread. What went wrong? First, it was thought that the new low-fat American diet would mimic the low-fat, high-carb regime of countries like China and Japan, which had very low heart attack rates. But the US food industry stepped in to provide us with low-fat foods that tasted good. It created delicious, highly processed foods including biscuits and baked goods prominently (and accurately) advertised as low fat, no cholesterol. This is the source of the 'empty calories' nutritionists decry – in whole foods, the sugars and starches are bound up with the fibre and nutrients, so when we eat whole grain rice, say, we get the entire package Processing removes the fibre (and hence, the nutrients) in order to make that rice easier and faster to cook. But as a result, all we get is the starch, and the calories – empty of the necessary fibre and nutrients.

In addition, the US Department of Agriculture's (USDA) diet pyramid was built on a base of the so-called 'complex carbohydrates' – bread, pasta, rice, etc. Like most Americans, I took that to mean that I could eat these foods in abundance and still live thin, healthy, and happily ever after. I was taught in medical school that the only bad effect of sugars was tooth decay. If you recall the seventies, you remember how healthy bread, pasta, and rice were made to seem when compared to the supposed evils of meat.

What have we learned since those days? A lot. First, the concept of dietary fibre as an important component of our nutrition was unknown at the time of Ansel Keys' studies. We didn't begin to appreciate the critical role of fibre until the 1970s. Even then, most of the attention was on fibre's effect on colon and bowel function. In 1980, Keys wrote a book summarizing his studies; in it, he suggests that fibre *may* have been an important variable not included in his earlier studies.

It turns out that the United States and the northern European countries with the high fat and high heart attack rates also had the lowest levels of fibre in their carbohydrates. By contrast, less-developed countries with high-carbohydrate, low-fat diets had *lots* of fibre in their carbs. In the 1990s, the Harvard School of Nutrition, under the guidance of Dr Walter C. Willet, looked at the correlation between fibre and heart attack rates. The finding: When people eat high-fibre carbs such as vegetables and unprocessed grains and flour, the danger of most dietary fat becomes minimal. Only saturated fat remains a predictor of heart attacks, and even then not a very conclusive one.

When the American Heart Association and other national agencies first issued their low-fat recommendations, most of the fat consumed in the United States was the unhealthy, saturated kind. Not much was known about the effects of other fats (olive oil, fish oils, peanut oils, etc.). Because even the experts didn't fully understand the role of fat in health, the recommendations were to decrease total fat intake. In response, saturated fat intake *has* decreased substantially. In fact, the total cholesterol of Americans has decreased even as we have got fatter. Why? Because we are eating less saturated fat and more of the good fats, our total cholesterol has decreased. But while our bad cholesterol is lower, so too is our good cholesterol, the kind that actually improves cardiovascular function. A third fat in our blood – triglycerides – is also higher, another ill effect of obesity. Triglycerides contribute to clogged arteries.

Finally, we've learned more about the differing natures of fats and carbs when it comes to putting on weight. Ounce for ounce, fats have more calories than carbs. We've always known this, but we've misunderstood the significance. We took it to mean that carbs are less fattening. In reality, the opposite may be true. When we eat fats, we become satiated. As a result, we know when to stop eating. Carbs, due to their effect on blood sugar level, stimulate further hunger, thereby encouraging overeating and obesity. Again, this was simply not known at the time when the low-fat, high-carbohydrate approach was adopted.

In the late 1970s, Dr David Jenkins, of the University of Toronto, introduced the concept of glycemic index. This measures the degree to which eating a particular food increases your blood sugar and therefore contributes to weight gain. One of the surprising findings was that certain starches such as white bread and potatoes increase blood sugar levels faster than table sugar does. The best intentions of the USDA and its pyramid turned out to be a diet based on sugars! It is the widespread adoption of this way of thinking that has caused the fattening of America. National guidelines that were created to make us thin and healthy actually made us fatter and sicker.

Understanding popular diets

What about the popular diets promoted to the general public over the thirty years since those guidelines? Initially, most programmes followed the low-fat, high-carb orthodoxy. The most popular was the Pritikin Diet. This regime requires severe total fat restriction. In recent years, Pritikin has liberalized its view of non-saturated fats. I admire the Pritikin doctors for their commitment to prevention of heart disease, which has included the successful promotion of exercise. But the problem with the Pritikin Diet, which its proponents acknowledge, is that it is hard to follow and requires a tremendous commitment on the part of the patient. Also, the high carbohydrate content of the diet can worsen cholesterol and triglycerides in certain patients. It definitely is not a diet for the general public.

In the early 1970s, Dr Robert Atkins wrote *Dr Atkins' Diet Revolution*, which shocked all by advocating the exact opposite of the low-fat gospel. He called for a diet high in saturated fat and low in carbs and was immediately denounced by the medical and nutritional establishment. The criticism was undermined by the fact that the diet seemed to work much better than the low-fat, high-carb American Heart Association diet. It was also attacked in part because Dr Atkins limited carbs so severely that body fat was broken down for fuel, causing a condition called ketosis. In otherwise healthy overweight or obese individuals, there is no evidence I know of that ketosis is a danger. It is, however, associated with a decrease of fluid volume and some dehydration, which can be a problem in patients with kidney problems or those on anti-hypertensive medications. Overall, however, the spectre of ketosis has been overstated.

The major problem I have with the Atkins Diet is the liberal intake of saturated fats. There is evidence now that immediately following a meal of saturated fats, there is dysfunction in the arteries, including those that supply the heart muscle with blood. As a result, the lining of the arteries (the endothelium) is predisposed to constriction and clotting. Imagine: Under the right (or rather, wrong) circumstances, eating a meal that's high in saturated fat can trigger a heart attack! In addition, after a high-fat meal certain elements in the blood, called remnant particles, persist for longer than is healthy. These particles contribute to the buildup of plaque in the vessel wall. None of this was known at the time Dr Atkins developed his diet. But we know it now.

These adverse effects do not occur when the unsaturated fats are consumed. This is why we have strongly encouraged the 'right fats' in the South Beach Diet. They make the meals taste good while they actually contribute to healthy vessels.

The other major diet phenomenon of the recent past has been Dr Dean Ornish's plan. The Ornish approach is similar to Pritikin's. It calls for severe total fat restriction and liberal consumption of carbohydrates. He also emphasizes exercise and relaxation techniques. In several small studies, he has demonstrated improved vascular health as a result of his diet. The biggest problem that I see in the Ornish approach is one that he readily acknowledges: It is very difficult to follow. Another issue is its restriction of total fats. The polyunsaturated and monounsaturated fats are good for you and your vessels. So why not use them to make meals taste better? Also troubling is that in selected patients, the high carb intake can induce the prediabetes syndrome we'll discuss in chapter nine. Since at least one-quarter of Americans are predisposed to this syndrome, and it is present in more than 50 percent of those who have had heart attacks, it is no small concern. Ornish developed his diet when the deleterious effect of carbs was virtually unknown. Today, Dr Ornish is putting greater emphasis on high-fibre carbohydrates that will not reduce prediabetes.

I know and admire Dr Atkins *and* Dr Ornish. They have successfully fought conventional wisdom and have both contributed to the country's growing focus on heart attack prevention via improved diet and lifestyle. They have been criticized for the commercial success of their programmes but have persevered. Unless someone popularizes the science of nutrition, America will never get its difficulties with obesity and heart disease under control.

It is my purpose to teach neither low fat nor low carb. I want you to learn to choose the right fats and the right carbs. You will learn to enjoy foods that taste good, satisfy your appetite, and don't create hunger hours later. In this manner, you can develop the food plans that are best for you for short-term weight loss and long-term weight maintenance and optimal health.

MY SOUTH BEACH DIET

ELLEN P.:

I LOST 1½ STONE IN 2½ MONTHS.

My oldest daughter's bar mizvah was coming up, and I wanted to lose some weight – maybe 1½ stone or so.

My whole life I had always been able to eat anything and it never showed. I love sweets. Chocolates. My friends had always been jealous. They would say, 'How can you eat so much and still be thin?'

So it was a real shock when I hit 40 and all of a sudden, I started gaining weight. My metabolism changed, I guess. Anyway, I didn't really know much about dieting because I never had to. But when I looked around and saw all the weight-loss plans, I said there's no way I'm going to be super-careful about everything I eat, or drink any of those diet shakes, or any of that.

That's why this diet was perfect for me, because I never felt like I had to eat things I didn't like or leave the table hungry.

The hardest thing for me at the very beginning was cutting out all fruit. I love fruit and fruit juice. Plus, I'm home a lot with my three kids, and I'm always giving them snacks. At least twice a week my kids and I would buy slice-and-bake chocolate chip biscuits. I used to buy a lot of ice-cream, too. I'd sit and have a bowl in the middle of the day. Or I'd have cheesecake. Biscuits.

At first I didn't know if I could do it. When someone tells me, 'You can't eat this', it's almost like I want it even more. But this diet was actually pretty good from the start. My husband went on it with me, and it became almost like a little competition between us. You're not supposed to, but we weighed ourselves every day.

What I liked about the diet was that you really do lose weight right away, and you feel good about that. You can have lobster and prawn and steak if you're hungry, and vegetables, and you don't have to limit yourself too much. It wasn't even that difficult giving up the sweets. After a while you don't even crave the stuff. And if I was hungry I'd have a piece of turkey or something. Or cheese. I remember how my husband always had to have his bread. If we went to a restaurant he would smell bread the second we walked in. Once he went on the diet he would tell the waiter, 'Don't even bring it to our table. We don't want to be tempted.'

I was on the diet for 2½ months. And in that time I lost the 1½ stone. I know you're supposed to stay on the strict phase for two weeks only, but I stayed on it a few weeks longer. I wanted to make sure I would lose the weight in time for the bar mizvah. And even the strict phase wasn't so bad.

I guess I'm on the maintenance phase now. I'm not very strict about it, but I don't crave as much as I did before. I don't even look at ice-cream when I go shopping, and I used to want it so much. I used to eat sandwiches all the time, and now I'll have turkey or whatever wrapped up in lettuce instead of bread. I'll cut up leftovers like steak and put them into a salad. Before, I used to skip breakfast most days, but now I always have it, and it seems like that makes it easier to stick with the diet. I'll have an egg with turkey bacon and it satisfies me until lunch. Before, I wouldn't have any breakfast, but if I found some doughnuts I'd have those. I still have biscuits once in a while. But that's about it for sweets.

a day in the life

I started this book by describing, in a nutshell, how you would pass the initial weeks on the South Beach Diet. Now I'll back up and tell you in greater detail how a typical day will go.

Let's start with the first day of Phase 1. You no doubt treated yourself to a memorable meal the night before, but whatever carb-driven cravings you prompted came as you slept, with no further damage done. By the time you wake up today, your bloodstream is a relatively clean slate. The immediate goal is to *keep* it that way. We will accomplish that simply by not introducing any bad carbs into your system.

We'll begin with a two-egg omelette fortified by two slices of lean bacon, cooked in a spray of olive or rapeseed oil. You may yearn for your usual toast or bagel, but if you can get your mind off bread, the rest of you will follow. This will be your first test of the new regime. It may take a few days to wean yourself from the customary morning dose of carbs. But it's our goal in Phase 1 to begin reversing your body's likely inability to process sugars and starches properly, the condition at the root of most weight problems. To accomplish this, we need to cut off all carbs but the healthiest ones, meaning we'll have those highest in fibre and nutrients and lowest in sugars and starches – vegetables and salads only, in other words, at least for these two weeks.

This morning's combination of proteins (the eggs and lean bacon) and good fats (the oil and the bacon), will keep your stomach full and occupied with digestion. You won't have to contend with hunger pangs now or later this morning. It didn't have to be the bacon omelette – we could have gone with two eggs and some asparagus, broccoli, mushrooms, or peppers. That would have introduced some good vegetable fibre to the mix. An omelette with ham or low-fat cheese would have been fine too.

With this meal you can have coffee or tea if you like, with low-fat milk and sugar substitute. There are many sugar substitutes to choose from nowadays – I prefer one that's actually derived in part from a form of sugar, although it has no calories. Some diets prohibit coffee or tea because caffeine does intensify cravings somewhat. But you've got enough changes to contend with without having to give up your morning coffee too.

A phenomenon I've noticed when dealing with overweight people is how many of them skip breakfast altogether. Especially women, for some strange reason. It's not even necessarily an attempt to save on calories – they say they just don't like eating first thing in the morning. The problem is that this allows blood sugar to drop and hunger to increase over the course of the morning, resulting in powerful cravings for a lunch that includes carbs of questionable value – the very kind guaranteed to keep you overweight. So, especially if you're trying to fight off obesity, skipping breakfast is a bad idea.

Planning your meals

In Part II, we've provided a meal by meal, dish by dish eating plan for every phase of the diet. As you'll see, the array of breakfasts even in the strict first phase is varied. There's a frittata made with smoked salmon, for instance, and something we call Vegetable Quiche Cups To Go, which are made with eggs and spinach and, for the sake of convenience, can be prepared in advance and then microwaved at mealtime. We make liberal use of eggs for breakfast, which will alarm some people who have been taught to avoid them due to cholesterol concerns. It turns out that eggs contain no saturated fat and raise the good cholesterol along with the bad. The yolk is a good source of natural vitamin E and protein too. So up to seven eggs a week are permissible. By the second phase of the diet, we'll begin to reintroduce carbs, even toast and muffins, along with some cereals. Fruit, too.

Whether you feel the need for a mid-morning snack or not, you should be ready for one by 10.30 or so. Wisely, you remembered to pack a chunk of low-fat cheese. As I said in chapter two, the only low-fat foods I recommend for dieters are cheese and yogurt, because they're the only ones that don't add bad carbs to replace the fats. The sugar is limited to lactose – milk sugar – which is an acceptable component of the South Beach Diet. Not low-fat ones! They're convenient and they taste good. Most important, they do the job of filling you up with good fats and proteins. That means you won't arrive at the lunch hour feeling famished.

When lunch rolls around, you may have a salad – lettuce and tomato mixed with grilled chicken or fish, dressed in a vinaigrette made with olive oil. You'll also have water or a beverage containing no sugar. Another day you might choose grilled prawn on a bed of green salad, or a tomato stuffed with tuna salad. Niçoise salad is great, too. All these dishes can easily be made at home and, thanks to the trend towards fresh, healthy dining out, can usually be found in restaurants, too. Don't even think about limiting the amount you eat – the point of this diet is to eat well. Food is one of life's dependable pleasures, and it can be a wholesome one if you're eating the proper things. Accomplish that and you will be free to indulge in the improper things from time to time.

I hope you are beginning to see the pattern of these meals: They're all combinations of healthy carbohydrates, proteins, and fats. They are normal, everyday dishes intended to fully satisfy your hunger while depriving your system of the low-quality sugars and starches that have wreaked such havoc on your blood chemistry. You may have noticed that we're not discussing calorie counts, fat grams, or portion sizes. The South Beach Diet is designed so that you don't pay attention to any of that. One hallmark of this programme is its simplicity – life is complicated enough without having to analyse your food before you eat it. If you're eating the right foods you don't need to be obsessive over how much of them you eat. Since fats create the sensation of satiety much more efficiently than carbs do, you won't sit in front of the TV all night popping bites of steak into your mouth, though you can easily imagine snacking for hours on crisps or biscuits!

By the time you finish this book, you'll have a strong overall grasp of which foods you can eat freely, which you need to enjoy in moderation, and which you'll do without. You'll understand the principles of metabolism – not as a matter of academic interest but in a practical, nuts-and-bolts way that will give you a basic understanding of how foods affect your blood chemistry and how that then determines what you weigh. You'll actually learn how to control your blood chemistry and your metabolism through food choices.

Knowing how individual foods affect your internal workings will help you lose weight and maintain the loss. In the future, if you ease up on the diet and find you've gained a few pounds, you'll know how to undo the damage. The glycemic indexes of foods, which are explained and identified on pages 64–7, will be important tools to help you understand which foods contribute to obesity. But once you learn the basics, you'll have all the knowledge you'll need to eat properly. You'll find it easy to cook at home or eat out while sticking to the plan.

Changing your thinking

Okay, by now it's mid-afternoon, typically the first dangerous time of day, dietwise. This is when you might normally crave a sugar fix, owing to the natural dip in blood sugar and consequently, energy, that takes place about this time. This is when people tend to run to the coffee shop, the sweet counter, or the vending machines. Instead, you'll have nuts – let's say plain almonds (not salted or smoked). Nuts contain good, healthy fats, and they fill you up. It's possible to have too many of them, however, and undermine your weight loss. I recommend counting out 15 almonds or cashews or whatever you choose. Some people have told me they prefer pistachios, in part because they're so small that you can allow yourself 30 of them. Cracking and eating 30 pistachios makes it a more elaborate, and therefore more satisfying, snack.

Now it's time to begin thinking about dinner. Recent trends in fine food have brought us all towards something close to the South Beach Diet way of thinking – fresh vegetables, fish, and lean meats are the staples of dinner on our programme. So Phase I features dishes such as grilled salmon with lemon, roasted aubergine and a salad, chicken made with balsamic vinegar, or even marinated rump steak and mushroom caps stuffed with spinach. You could happen upon any of these on the menu of a good restaurant and be happy with them. And this is the *strict* phase of the diet! As you'll see in Part II, in the meal plans for Phase I, we rely on chicken, fish, lean beef, and plenty of vegetables and salads to go with them.

We strongly recommend that you have dessert after that meal. The second dangerous time of day is between dinner and bedtime. This is when all good intentions and strong resolve are challenged. Partly it's just the normal nightly routine – you unwind with a book or in front of the TV, perhaps in the company of friends or family, and the communal snacking habit kicks in. If you've got children, as I do, you've almost certainly got lots of temptations around the kitchen. Or it may just be that you've trained yourself to expect something sweet after a savoury dinner.

In any event, we've come up with two basic strategies for dessert during Phase 1. The first, and simplest, is to have some sugar-free gelatine. For people who love fruit, it may even make up for the loss of fresh fruit flavours during these two weeks. The other suggestion makes ample use of low-rat ricotta cheese. You can use it as the basis for a number of delicious, permissible desserts. This one is reminiscent of the Italian delicacy known as tiramisu, which combines cheese, chocolate, espresso, and ladyfingers: Instead, you take 110g (4 oz) of low-fat ricotta and stir in a few teaspoons of unsweetened cocoa powder, some slivered almonds, and a sachet of sugar substitute. It tastes great, and I guarantee that when you're done you'll feel as though you've had a real dessert. We've tried a number of variations on this – using vanilla or almond extract, lemon zest, or even topping the ricotta with sugar-free chocolate syrup and then baking it.

And that's day one of the South Beach Diet! By the time you finish the last bite of mocha ricotta, you will have already begun ridding your being of the cravings that pushed you into the growing (in every way) ranks of the overweight. Your blood is different from the way it was 24 hours ago: Healthier. Get through another day this way and you'll be even closer to your goal of weight loss, and my goal for you, of better overall health.

MY SOUTH BEACH DIET

DANIEL S.:

I FOUND THIS DIET EXTREMELY EASY.

I went to my doctor and said I needed a diet. And I said, 'I don't want you to give me pills.' I'm six-one and I weighed 19 stone. In my early twenties I was even heavier – probably close to 21 stone. I lost some of that, but then yo-yoed around with the rest. Physically, I'm in very good shape. Cholesterol, blood pressure, heart – fine. But I was feeling lethargic – unable to move around the way I should.

I go out to dinner a lot. And I was just loading up on a lot of bad things.

I am definitely a stress eater, so there were a lot of potatoes and pasta and stuff like that at night. Bread — I soaked it up.

For breakfast, I was always good. Lunch, I tended to be pretty good. It was late afternoon — snack-time — into dinner that was the problem. My afternoon pick-me-up would be a chocolate bar or biscuits or something. Clearly not what I should be eating.

And then for dinner — whatever I wanted. I put no limits on myself. Dessert included.

I would say that my downfall was starchy foods. 4 to 8 p.m. was the bad zone. An extreme day — a stressful day — would be different starting in the morning. I might have doughnuts or some kind of cake. I'd get an attitude that says: Hey — life's stressful. Might as well enjoy what you can.

I've been on this diet around a year and two months now. As I said, I've gone on a hundred diets before this one. A million diets. I've gone from very good results to just moderate. It's very easy for me to lose weight. It's been nearly impossible for me to keep it off. I'd lose for four months, six months. And then it would creep back up.

I found this diet extremely easy. I could reintroduce a lot of stuff into my eating after the initial strict phase of the diet. I found that, as we added foods back, I was able to live a fairly normal life, with some modifications of my own. The main thing is teaching myself that, after lunchtime, I cannot put bread, potatoes, or pasta into my system. So that's how I've lived the past year, not eating any of those foods after, say, 5 p.m. I can live without pasta and potatoes. But bread is the one I'm still weak for. And so I've just forced myself to do without it. At a restaurant I ask the waiter not to bring bread to the table. That's not to say I haven't had bread in the last year. But when I have had it — or potatoes or pasta — at night, it shows up as a stall in my weight loss. So there's a clear correlation between those three items and maintaining my weight.

On certain occasions — my birthday, for one, a few weeks ago — I went to a great Italian restaurant, and they made homemade pasta. I had a bowl and I soaked it up with garlic bread. It was phenomenal. But it was my birthday. I should enjoy myself on my birthday. I also had dessert that night. But the next night, and ever since that night, I haven't had any of that stuff.

For lunch or breakfast I'll have a little bread sometimes. Never later than that. And I don't feel denied at all. That's the difference between now and the past. There are times where I see bread and think: Oh, gee, I'd really love a piece. But I've taught myself to go without it.

chapter five

good fats, bad fats

A ll fats in our diets were initially condemned due to guilt by association. The dominant fat was saturated fat, and since there was good evidence that this fat was dangerous, all fats were presumed dangerous. To avoid saturated fats in the diet, a special type of polyunsaturated became popular: the trans fats. They are the partially hydrogenated oils in so many commercial products, including cakes, biscuits, and margarines. Unfortunately, they are as dangerous or more dangerous than saturated fats. They increase bad cholesterol levels and are associated with heart attacks and strokes.

An ever-growing body of research states that many fats do not have the adverse effects of the saturated and trans fats. In fact, evidence is building that the unsaturated, non-trans fats are actually good for us. Where Mediterranean oils are used abundantly, heart attack and stroke rates are very low.

The most impressive diet study ever reported was the Lyon Heart Study. Here, the monounsaturated fat rapeseed oil was used in a spread by one-half of the patients studied. All those in the study had already had heart attacks, but those receiving the good fat had a 70 percent decrease in subsequent heart attacks.

Another large clinical trial, the GISSI Prevention Trial, showed that fish oil capsules – omega-3 polyunsaturated fats – decreased sudden deaths. Several diet studies have shown that eating fish a few times a week prevents heart attacks and strokes.

Finally, a number of studies have documented that several forms of nuts that are rich in mono- and polyunsaturated fats help prevent heart attacks and strokes. This gives us a great variety of foods, oils, and spreads that can make our meals taste great while actually improving our health. So including the right fats in the South Beach Diet was an easy call, looking better and better as more good fat studies are reported.

Once we fine-tuned the diet, it seemed ready for a real test drive. We photocopied the rules plus some basic meal plans and a list of permitted and prohibited foods, along with a few simple recipes. We then began handing them out to our patients. Again, our top priority was *not* weight loss for its own sake — it was to improve our patients' heart health by changing their blood chemistry. We wanted a diet that would lower triglycerides (fats carried in the blood, which are necessary, but which in excess cause serious cardiovascular damage) and LDL (low-density lipoproteins, the so-called bad cholesterol). We were looking for a decrease in LDL both as a total number and as compared to the level of HDL, high-density lipoproteins, the so-called good cholesterol.

And we were also trying to affect one more thing, something that most cardiologists, unfortunately, have yet to give its proper due: the actual size of the LDL particles. When these are small, they easily squeeze beneath the blood vessel linings, narrowing the passageways with a buildup of fatty plaques that eventually leads to heart attack and stroke. Using the right diet, we learned, it is actually possible to increase the size of the LDL particles. As a result, they don't fit under the blood vessel lining as readily, and so won't clog the arteries and cause an emergency somewhere down the line. Most doctors don't yet test for this crucial factor. In fact, today most blood labs still don't have the equipment required to determine the size of LDL molecules. In the not too distant future, however, measuring for this will become standard procedure, as common as cholesterol testing is today.

Our secondary goal, of course, *was* weight loss, because when that occurs it's a sign that blood chemistry, too, is coming under control. I wasn't thinking that my patients would attain the lean, mean, low-body-fat physical perfection. And frankly, neither were they.

Almost at once, the patients who went on our diet began to experience positive results. Blood chemistry improved dramatically.

One patient, a man who lives in the Bahamas, came to us in pretty bad shape. Blood work showed high triglycerides, high bad cholesterol, small LDL particles: the triple threat. To make matters worse, he had stubbornly vowed never to exercise – it bored him, he said. And he refused to give up his beloved daily dish of ice-cream. With attitudes like that, he was heading for trouble. But on our diet his blood chemistry improved quickly – triglycerides down, bad cholesterol down, good cholesterol up. He never did exercise, either, and he *still* has his daily ice-cream. But as a result of the diet he's lost about 2 stone, and it's stayed off for five years.

Another man was in his mid-fifties when he became my patient. His blood pressure was high, just like his cholesterol and triglycerides, and he already had noticeable narrowing in his coronary arteries. To treat those problems, his previous doctor had prescribed the usual daily cocktail of pharmaceuticals that heart patients everywhere depend upon. We put him on the diet, and before very long his cardiac profile improved. His triglycerides, for instance, had been over 400, frighteningly high. After a month on the diet that number had fallen below 100, a normal level. And he had lost more than 30 pounds, which he's kept off. He's no longer taking all those heart medications.

Another patient should have known better – he is a physician, after all – but he was also an overweight diabetic who had recently begun suffering chest pains. He had undergone one angioplasty to open up an artery, but it had begun to close again. After our first consultation I put him on the diet. His wife did all his cooking and, understandably, she found it easier to eat what he ate rather than prepare two different dinners every night. She lost weight, too. This particular dynamic has been a pleasant surprise for us – couples losing weight and improving cardiac health together because one of them has to diet. It becomes a shared effort, and they help keep each other on the wagon. In fact, the doctor's wife lost more weight than he did. Between them, they dropped 5½ stone. And before long his blood chemistry normalized. His diabetes resolved itself, so he no longer requires medication to control his blood sugar and cholesterol. And his arteries stayed clear.

These cardiology patients lost ¾, 1½, 2, even 3½ stone within months. They started losing as soon as they went on the diet – within the first week. They kept it off, too. Best of all, they reported that the regime wasn't difficult. The few basic principles were simple and easy to remember, and the rules were flexible. Dieters said they never felt hungry or deprived. After a while they barely noticed that they were dieting.

Most of those patients, male and female, had what we call central obesity – excess weight concentrated around the mid-section. We physicians measure waist-to-hip ratio to gauge a patient's pattern of obesity: when the waist is bigger than the hips, it's a warning sign for present or future heart problems. The first part of the body this diet affects is the waistline – that's where middle-age fat tends to be stored, so that's where the loss is most noticeable. Our patients felt sleeker after just a week or so on the diet. This was very encouraging to the dieters and gave them the inspiration they needed to stick with the programme.

After years of prescribing failed diets, I was ecstatic with the results.

Before long, however, there was yet another pleasant surprise. We began getting calls and reports from friends and acquaintances of our patients who had heard about the diet, tried it, and were successfully losing weight. Our patients, we discovered, had begun suggesting the diet to family members, friends, and far-flung relations. Thanks to e-mail, it was spreading like brushfire. People who had no heart problems at all, even the youngest and most stylish denizens of South Beach, were hearing about the diet, trying it, and shedding pounds. We started handling a steady stream of questions from people we'd never met, long-distance calls in many cases, folks asking what the diet did and did not allow, or requesting recipes and volunteering stories of quick, painless weight loss.

Then reporters began calling. It's amazing how much space in newspapers and magazines is devoted to weight loss. It's become a spectator sport. In early 1999, we got a call from a news producer at a local TV station. They had heard about us and offered a proposition: They'd find a sampling of Miami Beach residents who wanted to lose weight and put them on our diet. The 6 and 11 p.m. news programmes would then track their progress daily over the course of an entire month. We were excited by the idea and confident of the outcome.

The series ran every day – during the sweeps period, when ratings are used to set advertising rates. Hundreds of Miamians went on the diet and lost weight. The station won the ratings race, moving to first place among nightly news shows, attributed in part to the South Beach Diet project. The station's news director termed it 'a huge success with our viewers', and reported receiving hundreds of phone calls and e-mails seeking copies of the plan. The South Beach Diet series became an annual event for the station three years running. Our programme became a full-fledged municipal endeavour in Miami – brochures explaining the diet and the recipes were handed out in supermarkets. They, too, reported high interest and increased sales of the items we recommend.

I've accepted many invitations to discuss our diet at medical meetings where cardiologists and others gather to discuss treatment matters, including prevention and diet. In the beginning, because I am a cardiologist, I expected to be grilled rigorously on my nutritional knowledge. Instead, it became clear that the diet was scientifically sound. Even better, doctors have begun trying the diet themselves and reporting back to me about their successes. So many doctors have lost weight and improved their blood chemistries on the South Beach plan that it's become known as something of a 'physician's diet'.

Many of the dieters who came to us through the TV news coverage have been in their twenties and thirties. One young woman, 2 stone overweight, had been trying to conceive for seven years. She tried the diet, lost the weight in just a few months, and then discovered she was pregnant. Though we were willing to take credit for this pleasant turn of events, it wasn't until about a year later that I discovered why the diet had allowed her to conceive. There is a condition called polycystic ovary syndrome that is a common cause of abnormal periods and infertility in young women. It turns out that it is due to insulin resistance or prediabetes. By reversing this syndrome with the diet, our patient's periods normalized and a successful pregnancy followed. She is now enjoying her lovely little daughter. Another woman, also in her thirties, an entrepreneur, put her entire company on the programme, and they all lost weight together. Many of the nurses at Mount Sinai have become familiar with the diet and, almost casually, have begun following it. They often stop me in the hospital corridors to give me updates on their weight loss.

We were encouraged by how easy it is to learn – and put into practice – the operating principles of this programme. For example, one of the TV news cameramen reported that he lost weight based solely on the information he picked up in the course of taping my interviews. A couple of years ago, I described the principles behind the diet almost offhandedly to a young colleague at a medical meeting. A year later I was pleasantly surprised to hear he had lost over 3½ stone on the basis of my shorthand explanation. That's become a hallmark of this diet: The basics are easily learned and applied, with no complicated rules, charts, or calculations.

A proven system

At that point we decided it was time to try and measure our results in a scientific setting. First, we tracked in detail the weight and blood test results of 60 patients who had gone on the diet. The results were encouraging: Almost all experienced weight loss, lowered triglycerides, lowered LDL cholesterol, raised HDL, and improved waist-to-hip ratio. I presented this initial experience at an NHLBI (National Heart, Lung and Blood Institute) symposium at the annual American Heart Association meeting. The director of the NHLBI acted as moderator of the session. I was experienced in presenting research at such meetings, but always in the area of heart imaging, my speciality. Now, I was out of my comfort zone and quite nervous giving a presentation on diet and nutrition. I feared I'd be deluged with hostile questions raising points we hadn't considered. Instead, the very first response from the audience was to congratulate me for having the courage to challenge the American Heart Association's low-fat orthodoxy. It became clear that many of the clinicians in that room had also had discouraging results with recommending low-fat, high-carb diets. I was relieved and very excited that we were on the right track.

We then conducted a study pitting our diet against the strict 'step 2' American Heart Association diet, which replaced the earlier, more lenient form of the diet. We allocated forty overweight volunteers to either of the diets, meaning that half (chosen at random) went on the heart association programme and half got the South Beach Diet. None of the subjects knew where their diet had come from. After twelve weeks, five patients on the heart association diet had given up, compared to just one on the South Beach plan. South Beach dieters experienced a mean weight loss of 13.6 pounds, almost double the 7.5 pounds lost by the heart association group. Our patients also showed a greater decrease in waist-to-hip ratio, suggesting a true decrease in cardiac risk. Triglycerides dramatically decreased for the South Beach dieters, and their good cholesterol to bad cholesterol ratio improved more than did that of the heart association group. We presented this study at the annual national meeting of the American College of Cardiology, where it was well received. We've come a long way since the day I decided to act as Test Subject Number One for the South Beach Diet.

At this point, the next step practically suggested itself: It was time to put everything we'd learned into a book and make what has happened here in our city happen across the country and elsewhere.

MY SOUTH BEACH DIET:

MICHAEL A.:

I LOST 2½ STONE IN 4 MONTHS.

I started this diet because my mother had seen a piece about it on the local TV news in Miami. She has heart disease and was concerned about my health – I was 36 at the time and I weighed about 18 stone. So as a Father's Day gift she made an appointment with the Mount Sinai Hospital nutritionist for me.

My food weakness was quantity. I'm not a big sweets person. I would drink a few beers, especially on weekends. That was tough to cut back on. I never ate breakfast, just coffee. For lunch I'd have a salad or pasta. But I snacked all day – whatever they brought into the office, I'd have. Pork rinds. Baked things. And a normal dinner – some kind of meat or fish, with potato or rice or pasta. A lot of high-carb foods. But big portions of everything.

It was even worse on weekends – I'd go out to eat maybe Friday, Saturday, and Sunday, and I'd have a drink or two with dinner. And restaurant food typically isn't the healthiest you can eat. I wasn't exercising at all, either.

When I met with the nutritionist, she said my habits weren't great but they weren't awful, either. It was just the combination of what I was eating, and how much of it, and the fact that I wasn't exercising. I had tried diets before, and had lost weight, too. Once I stayed on a diet for four months. But when I stopped, all the weight came back.

I finally went on this one, about a year ago, when I weighed more than I ever had. It had got to where my clothes no longer fitted, and I just was refusing to go out and buy all new clothing. That's when my mother gave me the gift of the nutritionist visit.

The first days weren't so bad. The nutritionist explained to me the initial, strict phase of the diet, and said I could stick with it for two to four weeks. I'm a real meat eater. So in the initial phase, which allows you unlimited amounts of lean protein, I was all right. What I gave up in carbs I added in meat, so I wasn't hungry. Eggs for breakfast with some ham in there. They told me to cut out the half-and-half with my coffee because of the fat, so I tried the no-carb and non-dairy creamers, and I just couldn't do it. That was one area I said I can't cut out. I'll use just a little.

That would pretty much hold me until lunch, which would be a small salad with a decent-size serving of cut-up ham or turkey or chicken. In the afternoon I'd feel hungry, so I snacked on low-fat cheese. I drank a lot of water. Dinner was chicken breast or grilled steak. And that was pretty much it. A small serving of vegetables, but not a lot. I was really trying to cut the carbs. No fruit at all for the first four weeks. Only water to drink. During this time, I also started exercising. Three or four times a week I'd walk on a treadmill here at home, 30 to 40 minutes at a time.

I ate the same way on weekends that I did during the week. If I went to a restaurant I'd have a small salad with low-fat dressing and then a steak. No beer, no alcohol, no dessert, no baked potato, no rice. I did the initial phase for four weeks instead of the two they recommended, because I found it very easy to do and I was seeing results. The Fourth of July came during the first week of my diet. We had people over and they were drinking and having all kinds of good stuff. But I stuck to my diet.

After that first month I started introducing carbs from the low end of the glycemic index. I'd have bigger salads, and I added some fruit back in, which I had really missed. I began having an apple or a pear after lunch. I found a whole grain bread in the health food section of the local market. It was very low in carbs, and some days I'd have a sandwich on that instead of a salad. I went on vacation that summer and did okay – I stuck to my diet pretty much, didn't gain any weight but didn't lose any either. When I came back home I went back on the strict phase, with exercise, too. On my next visit to the nutritionist we added some more vegetables, like sweet potatoes, wild rice, brown rice, squash, beans, and legumes.

After about four months, I was down 2½ stone. My initial goal was a 10 percent weight reduction in six months. I got there in four. My next target was another 10 percent, for a total of 3½ stone lost. From around Thanksgiving to New Year, I really didn't stay on the diet very strictly. Still, I did okay. I ended up gaining about 7 pounds over the holidays. In January, back to the diet – the strict phase – and exercising.

I've been on this diet almost eight months. I've never stuck with anything this long. I find it's not hard to do. You can do it when you're on vacation, or when you eat out. It just takes a little discipline and willpower. When people start digging into desserts around me, now and then I'll take a spoonful, too. But I won't have a whole dessert for myself.

I have another 1–1½ stone to go. I'm confident that by sometime this year – with exercise and the diet – I'll be there.

chapter six

hello, bread

Once you've lasted through the two weeks of Phase I and rid yourself of your sugar addiction, you are ready to begin adding more carbohydrates to your diet. By this time the insulin resistance syndrome has disappeared. The cravings for sugars and starches are virtually gone, too. It's a fresh start.

You'd think that the challenge would be to restrain dieters from adding too many high-glycemic index carbs too soon, but just the opposite usually happens: People are reluctant to leave the safety of Phase I and begin eating the kinds of foods that made them overweight in the first place. If it was bread or rice that made me fat, why would I want to start eating it again? I don't want to undo all the good I've just done. I certainly don't want to slow my weight loss.

Still, there are several good reasons for adding more carbohydrates. First, many are good for you, especially those in fruit. Even bread, if you choose a whole grain type, brings nutritional benefits. Also, it's important for dieters to enjoy their food as much as ever and have a varied array of dishes and ingredients from which to choose. People love to eat, and you can take advantage of that passion even when you can't eat every single thing you want with heedless abandon.

Of course, we add the high-glycemic index carbs slowly. Usually we recommend that you start with one piece of fruit a day, something that won't provoke a big rise in blood sugar. Apples are fine – their glycemic index is low, and there's lots of beneficial fibre in the skin. Grapefruit is another safe choice, as are berries and cantaloupe.

At this stage we advise patients *not* to have fruit with breakfast, however. Sometimes it will cause a bigger jolt of insulin if it's eaten first thing in the day, triggering cravings for more. And while fruit has lots of fibre, it also contains substantial amounts of fructose – fruit sugar. So save it for after lunch or dinner.

Another carb that can be added back in the early days of Phase 2 is cereal, either something eaten cold, like high-fibre wheat bran cereal (e.g. Kellogg's All-Bran), or real (not instant) porridge. (The South Beach Diet never requires you to weigh your food or anything ridiculous like that. But we'll counsel dieters adding rice back into their diets to eat servings no bigger than a tennis ball. And don't choose the biggest potatoes in the supermarket bin.)

In any event, if it's oat bran you want, we suggest that you have it with a sugar substitute and skimmed milk. Adding an egg, which contains protein and good fat, will slow the absorption of the carbs.

If you decide to have your new carbohydrate with dinner instead of breakfast, you can have a slice of whole grain bread at night without fear of doing any damage. But you can't have it at breakfast *and* dinner, at least not in the beginning. Here's the principle to adding more carbs back safely: Do it gradually and attentively. The goal is to eat more carbs again while continuing to lose weight. If you add an apple and a slice of bread a day and you're still dropping the pounds, that's great. If you try having an apple, two slices of bread, and a banana daily and notice that your weight loss has stalled, you've gone too far. It's time to cut back, or try some different carbs and monitor the results.

You'll go on that cautious way as long as you're in Phase 2, eating the most beneficial carbs and paying attention to how they affect you. I'm not talking about weighing yourself every day. I'm actually opposed to that – you can usually tell when you've put on weight, and if you can't your clothes will let you know. You should also be aware of foods that increase cravings. No two people will experience this phase the same way. Some dieters can have pasta once a week and experience no detrimental effects. Others have to avoid pasta but are all right with a sweet potato. Because we want a diet that's flexible and adaptable to your tastes and habits, you'll have to figure this dynamic out for yourself. Our goal is to help you arrive at a diet filled with foods that you love eating. These rules are sufficient for you to create your own version of the plan.

The most successful dieters, we've found, are the ones who try every recipe imaginable and take advantage of all the foods and ingredients permitted. They make interesting use of herbs and spices – especially the more intensely flavoured ones such as horseradish, hot peppers, garlic, cinnamon, and nutmeg. Our patient invented a new soup made with every green vegetable he could find.

Boredom is the enemy here. It leads people back to their old ways. So at every stage, it's best to make this diet as lively and diverse as possible.

The most effective strategy for achieving your goals is to make use of creative substitutions. This is one of the pillars of this diet – replacing bad carbs with good ones so that you end up eating the things you love, only slightly different.

We've already discussed the staples: whole grain bread instead of white, sweet potatoes instead of white, brown rice or wild rice instead of white, whole grain pasta. Those substitutions will take you a long way towards making this diet effective. But there are plenty of other tricks.

Here's a terrific one to take the place of mashed potatoes, which everyone loves and, of course, are absolute diet-busters. Instead of potatoes, steam some cauliflower, either fresh or frozen – it makes no difference. (You can even do this in the microwave.) Once it's soft, mash it with a little liquid butter substitute – I Can't Believe It's Not Butter! tastes terrific and has no bad trans fatty acids. Then, mix in a little non-dairy creamer, which also tastes good and is healthy. Salt and pepper to taste, and you've got something that quite honestly can compete any day with the real thing.

Back when we first started the diet, before the trend of 'wrap' sandwiches had swept through restaurants, we had some success getting patients to replace bread with lettuce leaves. They'd take sandwich contents – meat or fish, cheese, vegetables, even condiments – and roll them up in crisp lettuce. They found, to their surprise, that the bread wasn't as crucial a part of the sandwich as they had thought it was. The filling was what tasted so good and satisfied their hunger, much more than the bread. We also suggested lots of concoctions that came right out of the fifties – food stuffed inside other food, like tomatoes filled with tuna salad. We had people trying this with any vegetable large enough and strong enough to withstand such treatment: stuffed aubergine, courgette, and artichokes were big favourites.

We tried a few dessert tricks, too. People who love chocolate almost always love lots of it, but they don't realize how satisfying even smaller amounts can be. Instead of some big chocolate dessert, try strawberries dipped in dark chocolate (which has less sugar than the milk chocolate variety). A few of these and you're satisfied, but in truth you've had a relatively small amount of chocolate and quite a bit more fruit. We also told some people to slice bananas, freeze them, and then dip the slices in a sugar-free chocolate sauce. It satisfies any sweet tooth, again, with a small amount of chocolate.

Using the strategy of substitution you can continue eating things that other programmes would banish forevermore, including some of the delicacies listed here. First, though, you need to know exactly which ingredients require replacement. The foods and food combinations that follow can, with modifications, support your weight-loss efforts instead of slowing them down.

Bacon and eggs

Even recently, the prevailing view of nutrition would behold the classic American breakfast of eggs, bacon, hash browns, toast, orange juice, and coffee and easily pick out what's unhealthy – the eggs (cholesterol), bacon (fat), and coffee (caffeine) – from what's good for you – the potatoes (a vegetable), bread (nothing's more wholesome than toast, right?) and the OJ (all that vitamin C).

Of course, that view is wrong based on what we know now. That's what even physicians find most frustrating about science: What's praised as good today may be condemned as bad tomorrow, and vice versa. It's not necessarily that we were wrong then and right now. It's just that our knowledge is constantly growing, and along the way we sometimes have to unlearn what we thought was true.

Breakfast is a good example of this. Back before World War II, eggs were considered healthy – high in protein and other nutrients. Then, beginning in the seventies, when doctors first began looking into the ill effects of cholesterol, eggs suddenly became a prime culprit. You were advised to limit yourself to two or three a week, and none at all if you suffered from high cholesterol. Bacon, too, because of the saturated fats and chemicals used in curing it, was portrayed as not just bad but toxic. We didn't worry about carbohydrates as a category of food, and especially not about orange juice, which became a favourite health drink.

We now know that eggs are a perfectly fine food – it turns out that they raise both kinds of cholesterol, the good along with the bad, and they do nothing to adversely affect the ratio of the two, which is the number that really counts. The yolk contains natural vitamin E, an important antioxidant that helps prevent cancer and heart disease.

Even the bacon's not so terrible, so long as you don't overdo it. The coffee's acceptable too, with the same caution.

The rest of the breakfast, though, has got to go. The hash browns? We've already discussed how high the glycemic index of potatoes is, especially the white ones. And when a food is chopped into small pieces, it more rapidly yields its sugars and starches. Take a white potato, cut it into slivers, deep-fry it in some unhealthy oil – it tastes great but wreaks havoc on your blood chemistry.

The toast? You know by now how bad white bread is for anyone trying to lose weight. Each slice is worse than a spoonful of table sugar. If the label on the bread boasts that it's 'enriched', or 'fortified' you're really in trouble – manufacturers add nutrients only because the natural ones in the wheat have been removed along with the fibre. People today feel wise when they order wholemeal or rye toast, another triumph of marketing and labelling, because in itself the term 'wholemeal' is almost meaningless. The bread may have more nutrients, but the flour is still highly refined. That label does not signify that you're getting the entire grain of wheat, fibre and all, as you should – that's only in whole *grain* (granary) bread.

Did you decide, for health reasons, to spread your toast with jam instead of butter? The problem with that decision is that most jams are loaded with sugar. Butter (within limits) would actually be better for you, since fat slows the absorption of the carbs in the bread. There are better things to eat on bread than butter, but jam isn't one of them.

How about that orange juice? If it's processed and sold in a carton, you could drink cola and be not much worse off. There are good nutrients in orange juice, but you can get those any number of ways without having to take in all the sugar that comes along for the ride in processed juice. Fresh-squeezed is somewhat better, because it has fibre – the pulp – that slows the absorption of the fructose. We tend to believe that the sweetness of fruit and the sweetness of, say, boiled sweets, are two totally different things, but they are not: All the tastes we describe as sweet come from sugars. Fructose, the sugar found in fruit, does in fact have a lower glycemic index than table sugar. Mixed in with fibre, fructose is acceptable.

Without the fibre, it can hurt your diet. So eat whole fruit rather than juice.

Can you have your favourite breakfast and stick to the South Beach Diet? Yes, with a few modifications.

Cook the eggs in a healthy way, such as boiling or poaching. If you fry, use a spray oil – either soy, rapeseed, or olive – rather than butter or margarine.

Try using lean bacon instead of the usual kind – it's lower in saturated fat, and higher in protein than the regular kind.

The potatoes have got to go – there's no way to salvage them. But they can be replaced with cereal, especially rolled oats, which has lots of fibre and helps with cholesterol, too. Stay clear of instant porridge, however – less fibre, more bad carbs. Get the kind you actually have to cook for a few minutes, the coarser the better, and use a sugar substitute, not sugar, and skimmed milk (if you require any). Porridge oats may not be an even swap for those good home-made chips, but it can be an acceptable substitute. Some sacrifices must be made.

If you love the taste of orange too much to give it up, eat the whole fruit. That way you get juice, flesh, fibre, nutrients, vitamin C – the whole package as nature intended it. And I'll wager you won't consume three or four oranges at a sitting, the way you do when you drink a big glass of juice.

You can have a slice of whole grain toast, topped with some heart-healthy spread – there are several good ones out there to be found in most supermarket dairy sections. These are not the margarines of old, which contain those bad trans fatty acids that can harm your cardiovascular system.

The coffee is fine, too, with semi-skimmed milk and sugar substitute (if required).

Nowadays, of course, the classic bacon and egg breakfast is being overshadowed by its fast-food interpretation – the Egg McMuffin. In this meal we have to contend with the bad, saturated fat in the bacon. But the portion of meat is so small that it's not really a major concern, unless you're having two of these every day. As for the egg itself, it's probably not being cooked in the healthiest fat, but again, there's good protein and nutrients without dangerous amounts of bad cholesterol, so even this is permissible. The biggest problem, of course, is in the highly processed carbs in the white-flour muffin. If you have that plus the potatoes and fruit juice, you're having a high-glycemic load start to your day, ensuring cravings for more carbs before lunchtime. McDonald's is no health food emporium, but then no one who dines there is under any false impression. If you must indulge, either throw away the entire muffin and eat with a fork, or just order the scrambled eggs and bacon breakfast, hold the potatoes, hold the juice.

Banana split

It seems wholesome, as desserts go, but this one is a killer. Banana is fruit, true, but like most tropical fruits it has a fairly high glycemic index, up near pineapple and mango. So first we've got to replace it with strawberries or blueberries or raspberries, all of which go just as nicely with ice-cream. Along with the fruit, add some nuts – not the kind drenched in sugary syrup, but raw walnuts, almonds, Brazil nuts, or peanuts. They're fine for you and add some bulk and good fat. As for the ice-cream itself, there's not much you can do. True, it's loaded with sugar, which is no diet's friend. But it's also loaded with fat, meaning that once you eat it your hunger will be satiated. And you won't be under the delusion that you've been good, so you'll be less likely to think you deserve more tomorrow night. Whereas eating low-fat ice-cream or frozen yogurt has none of these advantages – the fat has been replaced with sugar, so it's actually worse for your diet, plus it won't be as satisfying as the real thing, and you might actually convince yourself that you've been virtuous. If you're going to break the rules, you should at least know you did it.

Cheeseburger

This may be the pinnacle of American cuisine – a cheeseburger, chips, and a Coke. You can't deny that it's delicious, and thanks to the fast-food empires we've built, it's the easiest meal to come by in the history of eating. It's also highly problematic, though not for the reasons you've been led to believe.

The average fast-food burger itself is something of a health hazard, due to its high saturated fat content and the grease in which it's cooked. Eating one a day is a very bad habit indeed, but as an occasional treat it can be accommodated into the South Beach regime. However, if instead of this you have a burger in an upscale restaurant, or better still at home, you begin to change it instantly. You can have a burger made from a good cut of meat, like sirloin, which is much leaner than common minced beef.

But what will you serve that burger on? The usual soft white bun is all sugar. It's improved just by throwing the top half away and eating your meal with a knife and fork. Even better is to have that burger on wholemeal pitta or sourdough bread instead of the bun. While sourdough bread is not whole grain, it has another quality that decreases its glycemic index: It is acidic. Acid slows down the stomach's emptying of food into the small intestine, meaning slower overall digestion and slower increase and subsequent decrease in blood sugar.

Best of all – see if you can live without any bread on it whatsoever.

Next, the ketchup should go – even if you don't use much, it's loaded with sugar. Tomato slices are fine. Lettuce, pickles, and onions are perfect. Mustard's great, and even mayonnaise, as long as you don't overdo it. Remember to use the regular kind, not the low fat. Regular mayonnaise is high in fat, but it is predominantly soya bean oil, a good fat. Salsa, hot sauce, steak sauce are all fine too.

The chips are diet wreckers, thanks to their starchy nature but also to the bad fats in which they're cooked. To improve the taste, some restaurants cook them in lard, which just increases the danger. Even crisps are a wiser choice. Deep-fried sweet potatoes are better still, cooked in a monounsaturated oil. Best of all: Find another vegetable – like a salad. But if you must have your potatoes once in a while, don't supersize them.

The other lethal member of this trinity, the cola, must of course be replaced with a diet drink at the very least, if you can't go all the way to water.

Replace your typical cheeseburger, chips, and Coke meal with a topless burger (removing the top half of the bun), a salad with no cheese, and a diet drink, and the carbs drop dramatically.

A peanut butter and jam sandwich

The least harmful part of this classic is the peanut butter, of course. It's a good source of monounsaturated fat. It contains resveratrol, too, the same phytochemical that makes red wine beneficial as a protection against heart disease and cancer. Peanut butter also contains folic acid, which helps you to metabolize homocysteine, a byproduct of protein metabolism that otherwise can harm the cardiovascular system. The drawbacks to commercially processed peanut butter are that bad fats – saturated ones – are sometimes added, and so is sugar. If you stick to all-natural peanut butter you'll be best off. Jam is like eating sugar from the bowl; even teamed with peanut butter it will jolt your pancreas into making more insulin than is healthy. And the bread you're no doubt eating all this on is the standard supermarket white – the worst thing out there. All together, this sandwich is more like a desert than anything else. Best bet: natural peanut butter on pitta or sourdough bread, with skimmed milk. Even with those modifications, this should be a special treat only.

Pizza and beer

I'll bet you can guess by now that the oil and the cheese on the pizza aren't the worst things it has to offer. Especially if it's good olive oil and light mozzarella. The crust is white flour, which *is* a problem. And the beer, of course, is nobody's idea of a diet drink – maltose, the sugar in beer, has a higher glycemic index than white bread. The insulin response to it leads to the fat storage in the abdomen that we call, quite accurately, the beer belly. But pizza isn't completely devoid of benefits: Cooked tomatoes (as in the sauce) are a great source of lycopene, a cancer fighter. Completely eliminate pizza and pasta forever and you lose two of the most palatable ways to serve this vegetable. If you can switch from deep dish to thin crust, you've made a difference. And if, along with the olive oil and tomato sauce and low-fat cheese you add some green peppers, onions, mushrooms, and olives, you've added lots of good, nutritious carbs that will make the dish more filling. In place of the beer, try a glass of red wine. Now it's a whole new meal: not quite health food, but better than take-out deep-dish pizza.

MY SOUTH BEACH DIET

KANDY K.:

I NEVER FELT THAT HUNGRY.

I read something in the paper about the South Beach Diet just around the time I decided that I needed to lose a stone. And it sounded like a reliable plan – not one of those crazy fad diets you hear about. The fact that it was invented by a cardiologist helped, too. So I started.

Carbs had always been my weakness. I love doughnuts. When you pass a doughnut place with your son and he wants one, you don't just order one lonely doughnut for him. It's more like: 'Well, okay – make that two doughnuts.' I don't really have a particular problem, but I do like that kind of junk.

The first two weeks, the strict phase, were somewhat difficult, because you are so limited. I thought, 'You know, this is not going to be as easy as it sounded.' Going to restaurants and not having bread was tough. But it was an easy diet, too, because you didn't have to eat certain foods at each meal. You could substitute. If you don't like this, you can have that. If you don't want cheese for a snack, you can have nuts. Which made it very easy to live with. It wasn't prepackaged foods like on some diets where tonight you must have this, and tomorrow for breakfast you have to have this. You can eat the things you like. That was definitely the good part.

And once you grew accustomed to what you could and couldn't have, and you knew the guidelines, then even the strict phase became much easier. I never felt that hungry. You fill up on the things you're allowed to have. So you feel all right. You adjust to it.

I lost about 10 pounds on the diet, but now that I started working with a personal trainer, and I've actually put back about 5 of those pounds in muscle. But I'm much firmer than before – muscle weighs more than fat. There are days when I still want to stop at the doughnut place. But now I say, 'Oh, no, no – I'm not going to do that again.'

chapter seven

it's not just what you eat, it's how you eat it

As we've seen, the equation behind most obesity is simple: The faster the sugars and starches you eat are processed and absorbed into your bloodstream, the fatter you get.

Therefore, anything that speeds the process by which your body digests carbohydrates is bad for your diet, and anything that slows it down is good. Digestion is simply the action of your stomach breaking food down into its components; anything that keeps food intact longer is beneficial for people trying to lose weight.

Keeping that in mind, it's important to recognize that the process of digestion begins even before you swallow your food. In fact, it starts the moment you start preparing it. Example: Raw broccoli is crunchy, hard, cold, and covered with a layer of nutritious fibre. If you eat it that way, your stomach has really got to work in order to get at the carbs. That's a good thing. Of course, apart from a cocktail party's crudité table, we almost never eat broccoli in the raw. First we wash it, then we throw away the toughest part of the stalk, and then we cut it up and boil it or steam it until it's soft and warm.

That's also a fair approximation of what your stomach does to food – through the combination of churning muscles and the potent gastric juices and acids it produces, your stomach physically tears food to shreds and partly liquefies it. Whether it's in a pot on the stove or in your stomach, the same essential process happens to the broccoli and everything else you eat.

In the case of processed foods, digestion begins even earlier – in fact, it starts long before the food hits the supermarket shelf. Consider that loaf of sliced white bread. First the wheat is stripped of the bran and fibre. Then it's pulverized into the finest white flour. The baking process puffs it up into light, airy slices of bread. No wonder your stomach makes such quick work of it. A slice of white bread hits your bloodstream with the same jolt you'd get by eating a tablespoon of table sugar right from the bowl! Marie Antoinette would have a hard time telling it from cake, and the truth is that there's not much difference.

Whereas real, old-fashioned bread – the coarse, chewy kind with a thick crust and visible pieces of grain – puts your stomach to work. It, too, is made of wheat, but the grains haven't been processed to death. You may even see pieces of bran there in the bread. It contains starches, which are just chains of sugars, but they are bound up with the fibre, and so digestion takes longer. As a result, the sugars are released gradually into the bloodstream. If there's no sudden surge in blood sugar, your pancreas won't produce as much insulin, and you won't get the exaggerated craving for more carbs.

This is crucial to understanding how your body operates: The more food is preprocessed, the more fattening it will be.

The good news, of course, is that you can control the glycemic index of your food in part, just by choosing how you'll prepare it.

Take a potato, for instance. An incredibly versatile vegetable. You can do a hundred things with it, from soup to vodka. And what you do with it determines how fattening it is.

The worst way, from the glycemic index perspective? Baked. The process of baking it renders the starches most easily accessible to your digestive system.

Slightly better? Believe it or not, that baked potato will be less fattening topped with a dollop of low-fat cheese or sour cream. The calorie count will be slightly higher, but the fat contained in the cheese or sour cream will slow down the digestive process, thereby lessening the amount of insulin that potato prompts your body to make.

(Still, don't think that when you're out shopping and stop for a quick baked potato at one of those franchise places that you're having a healthy snack. A baked potato in mid-afternoon practically guarantees that you'll be starving for carbs by dinner. You'd be better off having a small ice-cream or even a dark chocolate bar instead of that baked potato.)

Better than baked? Mashed or boiled, due to the difference in the cooking process, but also because you'd probably eat them with a little butter or sour cream, and the fat slows the digestive process. Even chips are better than baked, believe it or not, because of the fat in which they're cooked. Of course, the same is true of crisps, but don't be misled: None of these are good choices for someone on the South Beach Diet. The type of potato you eat is also a big factor in all this. Red-skinned potatoes are highest in carbs. White-skinned are better. New potatoes, better yet – in every vegetable or fruit, the younger when picked, the lower the carb count. If you must indulge, do so sparingly. And try sweet potatoes instead of white.

The fibre factor

How bad is white bread? Worse than ice-cream. If you're about to sit down to dinner and need to decide whether to have white bread with it or ice-cream after, go for the ice-cream – less fattening.

But of course, not all bread is white bread. A good rule of thumb is that the coarser bread is, the better it is for you.

These principles apply across the board: Whole and intact is better than chopped or sliced, which is better than diced, which is better than mashed or puréed. All of which is better than juiced. An apple, for instance, has got a fair amount of pectin, a soluble fibre, in its skin. So if you eat an apple your stomach has got to contend with the fibre before it can get to the fructose. Similarly, an orange has got its fibre in the pulp and in the white pithy stuff that clings to the flesh.

But take that apple and peel it, and then juice it, and you've got something quite a bit different. The micronutrients and the fibre are in the skin. With the skin intact, it may take you five minutes to eat that apple. But it requires just a few seconds to drink the equivalent in juice. And keep in mind that the glycemic index number is in part determined by the speed with which you eat and digest your food or drink. This is why diabetics having a hypoglycemic reaction quickly drink some orange juice rather than eat the fruit. And while fructose is preferable to sucrose, a big glass of juice acts a lot like a soda – a pure sugar rush. This is especially true of processed juice made without fibre or pulp, which for many people is the only kind they get.

The fibre delays your stomach's effort to get at the sugars and starches in carbohydrates. The fibre in vegetables like broccoli is cellulose, which is in essence *wood*. The nutrients are bound up in that fibre, too, so the stomach has to work harder to get at the nutrition.

Sugar stoppers

Fibre's not the only thing that gets in the way of sugars.

Fats and proteins also slow the speed with which your stomach does its job on carbs. Eating a little protein, or some fat – good fat, naturally – along with your carbs is beneficial. A little olive oil on your bread, or some low-fat cheese, is actually better for you than the bread alone. Pasta with tomato sauce and a chunk of Italian bread is an extremely high-carb meal. Such a meal eaten with some meat or cheese is better. Sitting down to a nice baked potato for lunch isn't such a hot idea. Having that potato with a piece of steak and some broccoli renders it better for your diet than a potato on its own. You'll actually make less insulin, and you'll reduce the cravings for more food in the hours ahead.

Here's a tip that will lower the glycemic index of any meal: Fifteen minutes before you begin eating, have a spoonful of Fybogel in a glass of water. It's true, this is normally intended as a mild laxative. But it's simply psyllium, which is fibre – nonsoluble fibre. When you swallow that spoonful, the fibre forms a slippery lump which makes its way through your digestive tract, clearing out anything in its path. When you take some before eating, the fibre gets mixed in with the food and has the effect of slowing the speed with which your stomach digests what you've eaten.

When we talk about diet we talk so exclusively about the things we eat that it's easy to forget how much has to do with the things we drink. But your body doesn't make that distinction – by the time your meal reaches your small intestine, it's *all* liquid.

In fact, what you drink is critical because it requires little digestion and therefore goes more directly into your bloodstream. If there's sugar in that beverage, it will speed into your system, prompting the burst of insulin that leads to cravings later on.

At one end of the drink spectrum, to no one's surprise, is water. By now we've all heard the health gospel that we need at least 4 to 6 pints of it a day. There's some question about whether we really require *quite* so much, but a good rule is to reach for water whenever you're thirsty. It's especially good for dieters because it creates the sensation of a full belly.

At the other end of the spectrum is beer. As discussed, it has a high glycemic index thanks to its main component, maltose, which is even worse than table sugar.

Wine, and even whisky, are safer bets because they're made from different grains, vegetables, or fruit. Not that whisky is part of any serious weight-loss effort, of course. White wine is better. Best of all is red wine, because it brings with it some significant, proven cardiac benefits thanks to the resveratrol contained in the grape skins.

It's no surprise that fizzy drinks are a major source of sugar, so I won't labour the point. Sweetened iced teas aren't much better.

Coffee and tea, of course, contain no sugar on their own. People have grown accustomed to hearing doctors advise against them, but I don't think they're all that bad in moderation. Some diets steer people towards decaf for the simple reason that caffeine does stimulate the pancreas to produce insulin, which is the last thing an overweight person needs. Still, the effect isn't all that great, and if a cup or two of coffee a day makes you happy, I think you should feel free.

Again, fruit juices are a big source of trouble, in part because we've come to associate them with healthy habits. They do carry nutrients, especially freshly made juices. But they also bring with them high levels of fructose, which can be the undoing of any effort to lose weight.

Because I live in Florida, the best fruit example I can think of is the orange. A patient of mine began showing symptoms of diabetes. His blood sugar was suddenly up over 400, not a good sign. He didn't have any of the conditions that usually are present with new diabetes, such as an infection or other stress on his system. I began quizzing him about any changes to his eating habits when he mentioned that a juice machine had just been installed in his office. He thought he was making a healthy choice by having two or three orange juices a day to replace the coffee he once favoured.

Cut the juice, I advised him — you're dumping too much sugar into your bloodstream. He switched to water and the diabetes immediately was under control.

Therein lies everything you need to know about fruit juice. If you were to eat an orange you'd get the same fructose as is in the juice. But you'd also be getting a lot of fibre in the flesh and pulp and membranes. Your stomach would have to work to separate the sugar from everything else in the course of digestion. In addition, you might eat one orange at a sitting, maybe two if you were hungry or they were on the small side. But peeling an orange is work, and eating one takes time.

Not surprisingly, ready-made juice is the worst offender.

Fresh-squeezed, because of the fibrous pulp and the superior nutrients, is somewhat better.

This holds for nearly all fruit juices. Pineapple juice? Just loaded with sugar. Grape? The same. All of a sudden, it seems, America's parents fell in love with apple juice and began giving it to their kids with every meal. From a sugar consumption point of view, this was a bad idea. The skin of an apple is actually quite healthy – the pectin is a good fibre that accompanies the fructose into your system. So eating an apple a day is still a prescription for well-being. But drinking its juice is not.

If you must have fruit juice, try just a splash of it in sparkling water – a spritzer, in other words.

When it comes to vegetable juices you've got a bit more latitude. But the health food store mainstay – fresh carrot juice – isn't on the approved list. As we've noted elsewhere, carrots have a high glycemic index. Beet juice is said to be good for many reasons, but it, too, is loaded with sugars. I've heard that tossing a banana into the blender along with a little milk and some berries, accompanied by ice, makes a good summer smoothie. But bananas are among the worst fruits in terms of fructose content. If you knew nothing about nutrition and were asked to guess which fruits and vegetables contain the most sugar, you'd probably fare pretty well. The sweeter the taste, the more sugar is present. Watermelon is bad. Tomatoes are better. Broccoli juice would be best, if anybody actually wanted to indulge in a glass every day with breakfast. So be glad that the South Beach Diet doesn't require a big glass of broccoli juice every day!

MY SOUTH BEACH DIET

KATIE A.:

I NEVER FEEL LIKE I'M MISSING A THING.

I've watched my weight since I was about seven years old. That's when my sister and I spent a summer visiting my grandmother in Pennsylvania, and we ate all the processed and packaged foods she had in the house –

and she didn't cook. She owned a business, and to keep us busy she'd give us money so we'd scoot down to the sweet shop My sister and I came back home from that summer looking like roly-polys.

I've been battling with my weight ever since. You name the diet, I've been on it. I even found a doctor who gave me injections to perk up my thyroid gland so I'd lose weight. I ended up with Graves' disease. I was on Weight Watchers, too. And, yes, I did lose the weight, and I got the badge and all that jazz. But you know what happens? You become so obsessed with food, and you're thinking so much in terms of categorizing your food — I mean: How many breads? How many fruits? How many this or that? You find that you're thinking about food 24–7!

My hang-up was carbs and sweets. I was working the evening shift at the hospital back then, so I didn't get to bed till 4 a.m. I'd start eating while still on duty because the patients were always getting biscuits and sweets. When you got a little tired, you saw everybody else sitting around snacking. You weren't necessarily hungry, even, just tired, so you went for the food. Then, I'd get home and I'd feel guilty about all the junk I ate at work. I'd say: Well, now you've got to eat something healthy. So I'd have dinner, and *then* I'd go to bed. All my eating was done between 3 in the afternoon and maybe 3 in the morning. I'd get up for work and only have coffee for breakfast — and come to work on the 3-to-11 shift. I knew that you weren't supposed to eat after 8 o'clock at night. But that shift puts you on an abnormal clock. It was crisps, and pretzels, and all of that. Banana chips *and* sweets — and biscuits and cake. Bread. Rice. That was it. And in my mind I said: Well, I'm not eating *that* much. Because I was grazing. A little at a time. I was also a tremendous caffeine drinker back then. I was drinking a six-pack of fizzy drinks every day — Diet Coke, or Diet Pepsi. But it definitely was not caffeine-free, and I learned later that the caffeine was an appetite stimulant for me.

I didn't gain it all at once — the pounds just started to creep on. Until one day, my mother was walking behind me at the shops, and she caught up and said, 'You know something? You're starting to *waddle*.'

That did it. That was two years ago, when I went on this diet. I've lost 2 stone since then, and I've kept it off. The best thing about this diet is that it is easy to stick to. It's even flexible. For instance: I cheated almost from day one. Maybe not during the first two weeks, the strict phase. But after that. You could have nuts, let's say, but you were supposed to count out just 30 of them as a portion. Well, some nights I didn't count.

But beyond that, I've stuck with it, unlike all those other diets I tried. I haven't had a piece of bread in two years. Not a grain of rice, either. It's a self-control issue. But at the same time, I don't feel as though I'm denying myself. There's plenty that I can eat on this diet. And I have lots of positive results that keep me going. I know now that I can go into a store and I won't be reaching for that size 18. I'm now between a 12 and a 14, and I'm comfortable with that.

I've been able to stick to this diet so well that about a year ago I confessed to the nutritionist at Mount Sinai that I hadn't had an apple or any other fruit in over a year. And she got all over my case. 'Katie, you should know better,' she said. Anyway, I'm eating every kind of fruit now. Lots of vegetables, lots of fruits, lots of salads. But I know a lot more about what I eat than I did before. Like, people don't realize that the MSG (monosodium glutamate) in their Chinese food is made from beets, which contain a *lot* of sugar. Or that carrots have a high glycemic index, too. I used to eat a lot of carrots, especially when I was trying to lose weight. I even travelled with little bags of them. So I was shocked to learn that carrots have so much sugar in them. You don't realize that those carrots, or those onions, just turn right into sugar that gets stored in your body as fat.

Lately I actually gained a few pounds back – I'll be honest with you – because I cheated with those nuts. I'm into cashews now, but I've done the whole gamut. I've done peanuts. And almonds. Again, you don't realize that there's sugar in nuts, too. Pistachios are wonderful on this diet, because you can have only 15 almonds but 30 pistachio nuts, because they're so small. And I think I've begun to overdo it with the pistachios, and I may have put a few pounds back on. But I don't even get on the scales anymore. I go by how I feel in my clothing. Because I don't want to do a number on my head with weighing myself every day. If I feel like I'm getting too carried away with the nuts, I back off. And I drop a few pounds. Just recently I found a baker who makes sugar-free cheesecake. I buy it and cut it into very small portions. Then, when I get a yen for it – it's not every night, it might be two or three times a week – I'll just go ahead and take a piece and defrost it. It's something that I can have. It's enough. And so I never feel like I'm missing a thing.

chapter eight

how eating makes you hungry

How eating makes you *what*?

Weren't you always under the impression that eating is what *satisfies* hunger?

Well, it is and it isn't. Eating does put an immediate end to hunger. But some foods also create new cravings by making you hungrier than you would be if you hadn't eaten them.

This isn't just a theory, or a matter of perception.

Dr David S. Ludwig is the head of the obesity programme at Children's Hospital in Boston, a physician who also teaches at Harvard Medical School. He is doing some of the medical world's most important research into the root causes of our weight problems. Ludwig recently studied how the breakfast eaten by some obese teenagers influenced their hunger levels hours later.

Three groups of overweight adolescents were fed breakfasts of identical calorie counts. One group's meal was 20 percent fat, 16 percent protein, and roughly two-thirds carbs, but the good kind – steel-cut porridge oats, meaning the flakes were large and the kernel of the oat was unprocessed, and so the fibre was intact. The second group also had a two-thirds-carbs breakfast, but they were served *instant* porridge, where the fibre has been stripped away to permit shorter cooking time.

The third group's meal was identical to a typical South Beach Diet breakfast – vegetable omelettes.

After breakfast, members of all three groups were instructed to eat anything they wanted for the next five hours.

The subjects who had the bad carb breakfast – the instant porridge group – ate the most during that five-hour period. They also reported feeling the strongest hunger pangs.

The teenagers who had the steel-cut porridge oats felt less hunger and ate less than the instant porridge group during the post-breakfast hours.

The group who had the vegetable omelettes – the low-carb meal – reported the lowest sensation of hunger and ate the smallest amount during the five hours after breakfast.

This is one of several recent studies testing the theory that eating bad carbs makes you hungrier, and that on a diet of good carbs and good fats (the vegetable omelette combines both) you'll want less food later. I'll explain exactly why this happens, but for now I want to emphasize what all the studies show: Eating bad carbohydrates – especially highly processed ones – creates cravings for more bad carbs, which ultimately is responsible for our epidemic of obesity. It's hard to overstate the connection between bad carbs and bad nutritional and cardiac health.

In another diet and hunger study, subjects who ate whole fruit reported less hunger than those who ate purée of the same fruit, and those who ate purée had fewer cravings than those who just drank the juice. In various other research projects, scientists found that eating beans causes less hunger than eating potatoes; raw carrots cause less hunger than cooked ones; foods containing whole grains cause less hunger than those containing cracked grains; ordinary rice causes less hunger than the instant variety.

There's a term for the basic physiological response to food that's behind all these findings: reactive hypoglycemia.

I will describe exactly what that means. But before I tell you, let me show you.

For years, every day at around 3 or 4 in the afternoon, I'd find myself running out of steam – weak, sleepy, sometimes even light-headed. Without thinking, I'd make a run for the doctors' lounge, where I would ingest a bran muffin and a cup of coffee. I actually thought that since the muffin was labelled low fat, it was healthy. In fact, the word *bran* was there mainly to keep people from examining the ingredients closely and realizing that the muffin was just a fairy cake in disguise. Even physicians were lulled into a false sense of security – the fat in the muffin may have been low, but the carbs it contained contributed quite a bit of fat to my waistline.

Having finished my snack, I instantly felt better. So give my body credit for knowing exactly what it needed: Carbs. *Sugar.* My body knew this because it detected that the level of glucose – the form sugar takes in our bloodstreams – had fallen too low. Glucose is a form of chemical energy that our brains in particular need on a constant basis in order to function properly. Without enough, we'd grow dizzy, faint, and eventually go into a coma and die. Diabetes is the body's inability to turn food into usable forms of energy; this is why without synthetic insulin, type 1 diabetics would not live for long.

So my brain detects hypoglycemia – too-low blood sugar – and my body reacts (hence the name reactive hypoglycemia) by creating the cravings that drove me, and maybe you, too, towards the nearest carbohydrate fix.

How carbs work

As we've already said, carbohydrates are contained in a vast and varied array of foods, everything from the most virtuous vegetable to the most decadent treat. All carbs contain sugars. These sugars, though, exist in several different forms and go by a variety of names, including maltose (in beer), sucrose (table sugar), lactose (in dairy), and fructose (as found in fruit).

Despite that similarity, no one who has ever craved a sugar doughnut has been satisfied by broccoli. The opposite might also be true, though it's difficult to find people who suffer from insatiable cravings for green vegetables.

It's easy to tell by taste which carbs are highest in sugars, and which yield their sugars most readily. It probably comes as no surprise that a milk chocolate bar gives up its sugars more freely than one made of dark chocolate, or a pineapple yields its sweetness faster than a grapefruit, or a slice of supermarket white bread produces blood sugar faster than a piece of Ryvita. The more sugar there is, and the faster it's released, the more acutely we sense that sugar 'rush' – the relief that courses through our bloodstream as we heed the call for carbs. Internally, though, our bodies treat all carbs in basically the same way – digestion is in large part the process by which our bodies extract the sugars from carbohydrates and turn them into fuel, which we either burn or store. Burning the fuel is good – that means we're active enough to make efficient use of the food we eat. Storage of a little fuel is all right, but anything more than that is not so good. You know that excess stored fuel by another term: body fat.

The job of carbohydrate digestion starts in our mouths, when we chew the food into bits and our saliva begins the chemical process of separating each mouthful into its components. In our stomachs, the food is further shredded by the organ's muscular contractions and gastric acids. Our bodies want to get at the sugars contained in carbs, but this happens at varying speeds, depending on certain factors. Essentially, the less encumbered these sugars are by other substances, the faster they enter our bloodstreams.

Carbs' competitors

Which substances get in our bodies' way? Fibre is the major factor that slows the absorption of sugar. That's the reason the highly processed oatmeal was worse, diet-wise, than the steel-cut variety – the latter had all the fibre still intact, and so before the stomach could get to the sugars in the oatmeal, it had to separate them from the fibre. Once isolated, the fibre passes undigested through your system; its dietary importance comes from its ability to slow digestion down. It's an obstacle to digestion – a good one.

This was demonstrated not long ago in a scientific study in which half the subjects were given the fibre known as psyllium (you probably know it better as Fybogel) 15 minutes before lunch. The other half had lunch without the psyllium first. In the hours after the meal, the fibre group reported less hunger than the others. As the day wore on they ate less, too. The reason is simple: In their stomachs, the psyllium mixed in with what they ate and drank and slowed down the digestion. Slower digestion of carbs, less insulin. Less insulin, less dramatic drop in blood sugar. Less of a sugar rise and fall now, less hunger later.

Fibre isn't the only thing that slows the digestion of carbohydrates. Fat, too, slows the speed at which your stomach accesses the sugars you've eaten. That's why, in the study of overweight adolescents, the omelette breakfast created the least desire to eat more later. We have found other factors that slow the digestion of carbs and therefore benefit dieters. Acidic foods such as lemon and vinegar slow the speed with which your stomach empties, therefore cutting back on the rise in blood sugar. You can dress salads or vegetables in both and enjoy the benefit. Even sourdough bread, while not high in fibre, is acidic, and will improve any meal.

This is an important lesson in eating properly and losing weight on the South Beach Diet. This is why we call carbs containing fibre *good*, and why we also think of certain fats as good, too: Anything that slows the process by which you process the sugars in carbs is, by definition, good.

The body's response

Once the food has been liquefied in the stomach, it travels downwards to our small intestine, where millions of capillaries absorb what we've eaten and transport it into our bloodstream. Once there, it travels through our liver and then everywhere else in our bodies to be used, stored, or eliminated.

But let's continue to focus on the carbs. As we've said, they all contain sugar in one form or another. Even the starches are merely chains of sugars; digestion cuts the links in order to make the sugar molecules available to us. What we're concerned with here is the *speed* with which our bodies get at the sugars. It doesn't all take place at the same rate.

Once the sugars enter our bloodstream, it is the job of the pancreas to detect this and go to work – producing the hormone insulin in sufficient quantity to get the sugars out of our blood and into the organs where it is needed, or into storage for future needs. This is where diabetics run into trouble: They ingest the same sugars as everyone else, but without effective insulin those sugars remain uselessly circulating in the blood-stream. Insulin unlocks our tissues and lets the sugars in.

Fortunately, the pancreas can tell how much insulin is needed to do that job. If the body experiences a fast infusion of sugars, a lot of insulin is required. If the sugars are metabolized more slowly, the insulin is released gradually.

This is a crucial difference, as far as obesity is concerned: Fast sugar is worse for you; slower is better.

Here's why. When the sugars are absorbed slowly, the rise in blood sugar is gradual and so, too, is its descent once the insulin begins to do its work. The slow decline in blood sugar translates into less insistent cravings for more carbs later. You recall what I described as reactive hypoglycemia – the sensation of hunger caused by low blood sugar.

When the decline in blood sugar is gentle, the cravings are lessened.

But when your pancreas detects a rapid rise in blood sugar, it pumps out a correspondingly high level of insulin to do the job. That results in a rapid plunge in the blood sugar level. The insulin ends up doing its job a little too well – the blood sugar level drops so low that new cravings are created, requiring more quick carbohydrate fixes. In order to satisfy so many cravings, of course, we take in well beyond the nutrition we require. We overeat, and this leads to more fat, more insulin resistance, more hunger, and more weight gain – a vicious cycle.

Therefore, we can most easily stop ourselves from overeating by two strategies:

1. We can eat the foods (and combinations of foods) that cause gradual rather than sharp increases and decreases in blood sugar.

2. We can learn to anticipate hypoglycemia and avert it with the timely consumption of snacks. This one is crucial: It takes much less food to prevent hypoglycemia than it does to resolve it.

The third thing we all should do is learn which foods cause the most rapid rise in blood sugar. In the early 1980s, Dr David Jenkins led a team of Canadian researchers who devised a scale to measure the rapidity and degree with which a fixed quantity of a food increases your blood sugar. They called it the glycemic index. It lists most carbohydrates, from table sugar, beer, and white bread at one extreme to spinach and lentils at the other. On pages 64–7 you will find a sample of the index, organized by food type. You probably won't be completely surprised by what you find there. Anything made with white flour is high on the list. That includes most desserts, breads, and baked goods, of course, but also pasta. Instant rice is also near the top. Certain tropical fruits are fairly high, as are some starchy vegetables, particularly potatoes and other root vegetables. The king of all sugars, the one that increases blood sugar faster than any other, is maltose, which exists in beer. Now you understand what's behind the beer belly: The rapid rise of blood sugar caused by guzzling this beverage stimulates a corresponding rise in insulin production, which encourages storage of fat around the mid-section.

Knowledge and use of the glycemic index of foods is becoming widespread, but there's an important caveat which is crucial to understanding the link between carbs and obesity. You must bear in mind that the degree to which your blood sugar is raised depends not just on the glycemic index of the food but also on the quantity. For example, carrots have a high glycemic index, but they are fairly low in carbohydrate density. Therefore, you'd have to eat several handfuls of carrots to approximate the total rise in blood sugar you'd get from a single slice of white bread.

I have a handy analogy I use to explain this concept to my patients.

Think of alcohol. When we drink it, our blood alcohol level rises, and when it goes above a certain threshold, we feel tipsy. When it rises further, we feel drunk. We know that when we drink on an empty stomach, we get drunk faster. If, on the other hand, we drink while eating, on a full stomach, it takes more alcohol for us to feel the effect. This is because when the drinks mix with the food in our stomach, it takes longer for our bodies to get at and absorb the alcohol into our bloodstream, which transports it to our brain, creating that intoxicated sensation. The principle at work here is this: The more slowly the alcohol is absorbed, the less it affects us.

Now let's consider what happens when we eat carbs – bread, for instance.

If we eat white bread, we're getting no fibre with our carbs. That's like drinking on an empty stomach: Our stomachs can get at the starches without having to first separate them from the fibre. As a result, the bread is quickly turned into glucose – blood sugar – and causes an equally sharp rise in insulin, which brings about the dreaded acute rise and fall of blood sugar level, thereby creating more cravings later on. Eating white bread is analogous to drinking alcohol on an empty stomach; eating whole grain bread is like eating with your cocktail.

The fibre is the part of the grain not absorbed into the bloodstream from the intestine but excreted as waste. Even though it is not absorbed, fibre helps digestion in another, more commonly understood way. It helps your colon to function efficiently – the lack of fibre in our diets is why constipation has become a common problem.

Fibre, then, joins fat, protein, and acidity on the list of things that delay the absorption of sugars and starches. We need to include one or more of the above in every meal in order to keep ourselves from getting drunk – on carbs. By choosing the right foods, food combinations, and strategically timed snacks, you can prevent hypoglycemia and thereby control your weight without having to fight off cravings.

A final anecdote to illustrate this principle: A friend and patient who was in the first week of the diet rushed out one afternoon to play golf. He had neglected to plan his lunch so he decided to break the rules and grab a sandwich. As he played golf, several hours later, he began to feel weak and shaky and recognized this as reactive hypoglycemia. There were no permissible snacks available, so he found some sachets of sugar and guzzled them down. They relieved his acute hunger and they tasted great, too. He returned home and downed a bag of tortilla chips and a chocolate bar. This binge was due not to a loss of self-control but to his poor planning. Once the hypoglycemia struck, the consequence was preordained. Had my friend eaten tuna salad instead of a sandwich and had some low-fat cheese or nuts as a snack, both the initial hypoglycemia and subsequent gorging could have been avoided.

MY SOUTH BEACH DIET:

PAUL L.:

I'VE CLEANED OUT MY MEDICINE CABINET THANKS TO THIS DIET.

I weighed 16½ stone five years ago, when I went on this diet. Over the years, I had always struggled with my weight, and I tried lots of the diets out there. I tried Atkins – in fact, I had actually been a patient of his years ago, before he got famous. And so I tried his low-carb diet. I also tried some of the low-fat diets, the Heart Association-type programmes. I always lost some weight but I always gained it back.

I'm 73 now, and I was 68 when I started with the South Beach Diet. I had been a heavy smoker and then I gave it up, which is how I happened to put on all that weight. I wasn't a big sweets eater. But I loved all the rest. Bread three times a day, with every meal. And potatoes. Rice. Pasta. Of course, meat and so on – big, heavy meals. Once my weight hit its peak, I started getting some other problems, too. One day we found that I had diabetes. My blood pressure was high. My triglycerides were high. My cholesterol was high.

I began seeing Dr Agatston as my cardiologist, and we discussed how my being so overweight was contributing to my conditions. He suggested the diet he developed. And because I was no stranger to diets, I said I'd give it a try.

The first few days weren't exactly easy. I wouldn't say you feel bad, but definitely different. A little off. You're hungry because you're not following your normal eating patterns. But after those first 3 days, it suddenly seemed easier. I wasn't really going hungry. I ate a ton of vegetables during that strict phase, and a lot of meat and fish and cheese, too. A lot of white meat chicken and turkey. But no bread or pasta or even fruit.

After the first two weeks, I started adding things back into my diet. I had some fruit, although to be honest, when I had a little fruit I wanted more. It was easier in a way to just go without fruit altogether.

I never did add any potatoes back to my diet – I just didn't miss them enough to want them, I guess. And maybe it's easier for me to have none than a little. I do like pasta, and so I'll have that every once in a while – say, every few weeks I'll have a dish. Rice, less so, though I'll have that occasionally, too. I have gone back to eating bread. I'll have it just about every day now, and two or three pieces. And I drink red wine – two glasses a day.

It took me about a year, but I went from 16½ down to 12 stone on this diet. 4½ stone in 50 weeks. And for the past four years I've been maintaining this weight pretty easily. Once it crept up again, to 12½, so I just went back on the Phase I diet and I got back down to 12 pretty fast.

The best part, though, is that I've cleaned out my medicine cabinet thanks to this diet. I stopped taking the diabetes medicine because it cleared up. Blood pressure medicine – gone. I was taking a statin for my cholesterol, but now I've even thrown that away.

THE GLYCEMIC INDEX

The following table lists the glycemic index of many of the foods you're likely to encounter in your daily life. The choices are grouped by type of food, then arranged alphabetically.

A food's glycemic index is the amount that it increases your blood sugar level compared to the amount that the same quantity of white bread would increase it.

The foods with the lower numbers will cause your blood sugar to rise then fall more slowly that the foods with higher numbers will. Numerous studies have also shown that low-glycemic foods satisfy your hunger longer and minimize your food cravings better.

In Phase I of the South Beach Diet, you should only choose foods with a low glycemic index. Later on, after you've gone through the rapid weight-loss phase, you can start mixing in foods with higher numbers.

However, still follow the other rules of the diet; even though skimmed milk and peanut M&Ms have the same glycemic index, the milk is a much better nutritional choice.

BAKERY PRODUCTS	GI
Cake, angel	67
Cake, sponge	46
Cake, tart	65
Croissant	67
Danish pastry	59
Doughnut	76
Muffin (unsweetened sort)	62
Waffles	76

BEVERAGES	GI
Apple juice	41
Carrot juice	45
Grapefruit juice	48
Orange juice	52
Pineapple juice	46
Soya milk	30

BREADS	GI
Bagel, plain	72
Baguette	95
Bread stuffing	74
Hamburger bun	61
Melba toast	70
Multi grain bread	48
Pitta bread, white	57
Pizza, cheese	60
Rye-flour bread	64
Wheat bread, gluten-free	90
White bread	71
White rolls	73
Whole grain e.g. pumpernickel	50
Wholemeal bread	69

BREAKFAST CEREALS	GI
All-Bran	42
Cheerios	74
Cornflakes	83
Golden Grahams	71
Grape-Nuts	67
Mini-Wheats (wholemeal)	57
Muesli	56
Oat bran	55
Porridge, non-instant	49
Puffed Wheat	74
Rice Krispies	82
Shredded Wheat	69
Special K	54
Weetabix	77

CEREAL GRAINS	GI
Barley, cracked	50
Barley flakes	66
Buckwheat flakes	55
Bulgur wheat	48
Couscous	65
Millet	71
Pearl barley	25

Polenta	69
Rice, brown	55
Rice, instant	46
Rice, parboiled	48
Rice, white	58
Rice, wild	57
Rye	34
Taco shells	68
Tapioca, boiled with milk	81
Wheat kernels	41

SWEET BISCUITS	GI
Biscotti	79
Digestives	58
Shortbread	64
Wafer biscuits	77

SAVOURY BISCUITS	GI
Rice cakes	77
Ryvita	67
Water biscuits	65

DAIRY FOODS	GI
Milk, chocolate, artificially sweetened	24
Milk, semi-skimmed	34
Milk, skimmed	32
Milk, whole	27
Ice-cream	61
Ice-cream, low-fat	50
Yogurt, low-fat, artificially sweetened	14
Yogurt, low-fat, fruit-flavoured	33

FRUIT AND FRUIT PRODUCTS	GI
Apples	38
Apricots	57
Apricots, dried	31
Apricots, tinned in syrup	64
Bananas	54
Cherries	22
Fruit cocktail	55
Grapefruit	25
Grapes	46
Kiwi fruit	53
Mangoes	56
Cantaloupe melon	65
Oranges	44
Peaches	42
Peaches, tinned	47
Pears	38
Pears, tinned	44
Pineapple	66
Plums	39
Raisins	64
Watermelon	72

PULSES	GI
Baked beans, tinned	48
Black-eyed beans	41
Broad beans	79
Butter beans, boiled	31
Chickpeas	33
Chickpeas, tinned	42
Haricot beans, boiled	38
Kidney beans, boiled	29
Kidney beans, tinned	52
Lentils, green, boiled	29

Lentils, green, tinned	52
Lentils, red, boiled	25
Lima beans, baby, frozen	32
Pinto beans	39
Pinto beans, tinned	45
Soya beans, boiled	16
Split peas, yellow, boiled	32

PASTA	GI
Capellini	45
Fettuccine	32
Gnocchi	67
Linguine	46
Macaroni	45
Macaroni cheese	64
Ravioli, meat filled	39
Rice pasta, brown	92
Spaghetti, durum wheat	55
Spaghetti, protein enriched	27
Spaghetti, wholewheat	37
Spaghetti, white	41
Tortellini, cheese	50
Vermicelli	35

ROOT VEGETABLES	GI
Beetroot	64
Carrots, cooked	39
Chips	75
Parsnips	97
Potato, baked	85
Potato, boiled	56
Potato, instant	83
Potato, mashed	70
Potato, microwaved	82

Potato, new	57
Potato, steamed	65
Potato, tinned	61
Sweet potato	54
Swede	72
Yam	51

SNACK FOOD AND SWEETS	GI
Chocolate bar, 30g (1 ½ oz)	49
Corn chips	74
Crisps	54
Dates	103
Jams and marmalades	49
Jelly beans	80
Life Savers or Refreshers	70
Mars Bar	64
M&Ms (peanut)	32
Skittles	69
Snickers Bar	40
Twix Biscuit Bars (caramel)	43
Peanuts	15
Popcorn	55
Pretzels	81

SOUPS	GI
Lentil soup, tinned	44
Tomato soup, tinned	38

SUGARS	GI
Fructose powder	22
Honey	58
Lactose	46
Liquid glucose	96

Maltose	105	Kale	<15
Sucrose	64	Lettuce, all varieties	<15
		Mange-tout	<15
VEGETABLES	GI	Mushrooms, all varieties	<15
Artichoke, globe	<15	Mustard greens	<15
Asparagus	<15	Okra	<15
Aubergine	<15	Peanuts	<15
French beans	<15	Peas, dried	22
Green beans	<15	Peas, green	48
Beetroot	<15	Peppers, all varieties	<15
Broccoli	<15	Pumpkin	75
Brussels sprouts	<15	Rocket	<15
Cabbage, all varieties	<15	Spinach	<15
Cauliflower	<15	Spaghetti squash	<15
Celery	<15	Young summer squash	<15
Swiss chard	<15	Sweet corn	55
Courgettes	<15	Tomatoes	15
Cucumber	<15	Turnip	<15
Batavian endive	<15	Watercress	<15

chapter nine

is it diabetes yet?

I see an awful lot of people with the condition largely responsible for the current epidemic of obesity and heart disease. You see them, too, whether you know it or not.

I see them in my examining room, of course, but I also see them on the street, at parties, at the shops, on the beach, virtually everywhere I look. They're very easy to recognize thanks to one unmistakable visible sign: central obesity – excess weight concentrated mainly in a rounded, protruding waistline, often on individuals with the face, arms, and legs you'd expect to find on someone thinner. It's commonly referred to as apple-shaped obesity – as opposed to pear-shaped, where the excess weight is distributed throughout the hips, buttocks, and legs.

People usually refer to central obesity by some cute euphemism – it's a paunch, a beer gut, a potbelly, a bay window. But to me it's a serious warning of unhealthy blood chemistry today and cardiac trouble ahead. In social settings, I have to restrain myself from urging people I've just met who fit the above profile to call me (or any cardiologist) first thing in the morning to schedule diagnostic blood tests. I've become something of an evangelist on this subject because the disorder is so widespread and dangerous, yet simple to treat using diet, exercise, and medication.

When I ask overweight patients about family medical history, they'll frequently tell me about a parent or grandparent who developed diabetes late in life, often in their seventies or eighties. 'But it was just "chemical" diabetes,' the patient will assure me, using an outdated term. 'He didn't even take insulin for it.' Sometimes they'll refer to it as 'sugar' diabetes, another relic of medical terminology. The patient has no idea that this late-occurring form of the disease in a parent is actually an indication that another, silent but potentially deadly condition is present – one that is setting the stage, internally, for his or her own future heart attack or stroke. The diabetes gene is passed along to all offspring. An early manifestation of the disease is weight gain during middle age – years before blood sugar becomes elevated.

But what does diabetes have to do with a heart attack or stroke? That's the question most people ask. Over the past ten years we have come a long way in understanding the connection. We now know without a doubt that they are linked: About half of all people who have heart attacks are found to be suffering from a condition that goes under several names. Metabolic syndrome is the most popular current term, but it's also been called insulin resistance, or syndrome X. We've known of its existence only since 1989, and we're still learning about it. For our purposes let's refer to it as prediabetes, since that comes closest to calling it what it is – an early stage of the disease. Unchecked, prediabetes today will turn into full-blown type 2 diabetes tomorrow.

By the latest count, somewhere around 47 million Americans – close to one in five – are estimated to have prediabetes. But the percentage of adults with cardiovascular disease who also have this syndrome is much higher; maybe half of my practice shows signs. Here's a list of the criteria, according to the National Cholesterol Education Program.

- High cholesterol
- High ratio of bad cholesterol to good
- High blood pressure
- Central obesity
- High triglycerides

To which I would add:

- Small LDL (bad cholesterol) particles

These are also the conditions that are closely associated with heart attack and stroke. Genetics plays a major role in determining whether you'll have these conditions. But so does improper diet. I'll try not to burden you with too much science as I explain the connection between heart disease and adult-onset diabetes. Trust me: It's important to understand this.

The facts on diabetes

Most people know diabetes as the body's inability to process sugars and starches properly. Your body digests a meal and converts all the carbs into glucose – blood sugar. It then becomes the job of your pancreas to detect this sudden infusion of glucose and, in response, produce the hormone insulin. The insulin is needed to allow your body's various organs – brain, muscles, liver, and so on – to extract the glucose from your bloodstream and either use it at once or store it for future use. The body's need for sugar is constant – without it in sufficient quantities you will become dizzy, faint, go into a coma, and before long, die.

Imagine that each cell in your body has a lock on it, and insulin is the only key that fits. If the cells remain locked, the sugars can't enter, and they remain circulating uselessly in your bloodstream, where they do you no good and cause considerable harm.

But what most people don't realize is that diabetes isn't just about how we process sugars: It's also the inability to properly process the fats we eat.

When we eat fats, whether from flesh, vegetable oils, or dairy products, it is also insulin's job to transport the fatty acids (the basic component of fats) from the bloodstream into the body's tissues, where they belong, to be used immediately for fuel or stored for future use in the form we know as triglycerides.

In fact, diabetes can be seen as the body's inability to manage its fuel supply well. Obesity, too, is just a matter of bad fuel management, due to a combination of genetics and lifestyle. Our bodies are designed to store excess energy (which we call calories) for a very good reason: For most of humanity's existence, securing a steady and sufficient supply of food has been our biggest, most important challenge. Feast or famine prevailed and, to adapt, our bodies would save the energy from today's feast, knowing that tomorrow it would need to burn saved fuel in order to survive. That's why this particular brand of obesity concentrates the fat in the midsection – it leaves the extremities lithe and muscular, for ease of manual labour and, especially, flight. Advanced civilization has done a great deal to eradicate famine, but at the expense of our waistlines and our cardiovascular systems, which now suffer from the fact that we store fat we no longer need. We'd be better off if our bodies eliminated excess energy as if it were waste, but they don't.

This is exacerbated by the physiology of the fat cell. When we gain weight, we're not creating new fat cells — their number remains constant from childhood. No, what happens is that the fat cells themselves get fat. That's why in overweight people the insulin has trouble attaching to the fat cells — they've grown too big. As a result, when an overweight person overeats, it's like trying to fill a gas tank that's already at capacity — the excess spills over. In your body, that means the sugars and fats circulate in your blood longer than they should. When your body cannot properly transfer the glucose and fatty acids from your bloodstream into your tissues, it's the beginning of trouble. Left untreated, serious cases of diabetes would be fatal.

But there are *two* types of diabetes, and these differ in important ways.

Juvenile (or type 1) diabetes usually strikes during childhood or adolescence. It's caused by some damage that's been done to the pancreas — possibly by a virus. As a result, the organ produces too little insulin to do the job of getting sugars and fats from the bloodstream into the proper tissues. It's an incurable disease so far and can be treated only by replacing the insulin with daily insulin injections. That's why eating carefully and measuring blood sugar level are so important to a diabetic's well-being and why insulin is such a lifesaving drug.

We don't even have a proper name yet for the other form of this disease; hence its working title: type 2 diabetes. This is also called adult-onset diabetes, because that's when it usually shows up. As we've said, there's no virus to blame, just who we are (genetics) and what we eat. A surprisingly large percentage of us are genetically predisposed to diabetes of this kind. But the predisposition is just that — the *potential* for diabetes — until poor diet and lack of exercise do their damage. We can't control our genes. But if you can keep from making bad food choices, you can prevent this form of diabetes.

Both these diseases go by the same name, but the causes are opposite. Juvenile diabetes is a result of the pancreas's inability to produce insulin. In type 2, your pancreas is fully functional and is actually making *too much* insulin. We discussed this earlier: When you carry excess body fat, you make it difficult for insulin to do its job. So the blood sugar level doesn't lower as quickly as it should, prompting your pancreas to pump out even more insulin in order to unlock your cells and let the glucose in. Your pancreas sends out insulin until finally it overshoots the mark, which is why the blood sugar level goes so low. It's the high level of sugar in the bloodstream and then the rapid plunge (when you finally produce enough insulin) that causes your sharp food cravings. Which in turn causes you to eat more carbs, and so the vicious cycle goes around and around.

All the above is fine and good as an explanation for why obesity makes you overeat, and why eating carbs, rather than satisfying your hunger, makes you hungry for more. But we still haven't answered this question: What do obesity and type 2 diabetes or prediabetes have to do with heart trouble?

Effects on the heart

It starts with that central obesity. Your expanding mid-section is not due to an increase in the *number* of fat cells in there. No, when you're overweight, the number of cells remains more or less constant, but each cell increases in size. In other words, the fat cells themselves grow fat. When these cells expand, the insulin has trouble attaching to them properly and unlocking them. That's why, if you weigh too much, the sugar and fat levels in your bloodstream rise higher than they should. The insulin key takes longer to open the lock.

That in turn brings about several other conditions of the blood, all of which are further symptoms of type 2 diabetes and even prediabetes, signs that can be seen only by a doctor. They're a familiar list if you've been paying attention to health news over the past decade: High blood pressure, high triglycerides, high total cholesterol, high ratio of bad cholesterol to good, and the relatively unknown but critical matter of too-small bad cholesterol particles.

When insulin isn't working properly, it takes longer than it should to store the fat you just ate. Because of that delay, your liver is being flooded with fatty acids. In response to that, the organ emits harmful particles that deposit fat and cholesterol in the blood vessels of your heart. Future blockages, in other words.

So this, then, is the link between obesity and heart disease. The danger isn't the carbs or the sugars in themselves. It's how they affect your body's ability to process fats. Eating too many jam doughnuts may not cause a heart attack. But it can and does create the conditions that will lead to one. Obesity itself doesn't damage your cardiovascular system. It's just the number-one sign of an unhealthy blood profile, which will someday almost certainly curtail your good health, and maybe your life.

Today, alarmingly, we're seeing type 2 diabetes in young adults and even in adolescents. It's not that we're congenitally less healthy than previous generations. But our habits are much worse. Gym memberships and home treadmills are staples of middle-class life, but the truth is that we perform less physical activity than our parents and grandparents did. Maybe their jobs required more exertion, or they enjoyed fewer labour-saving devices. Perhaps they just walked a lot more than we do.

This lack of exercise extends even to the youngest among us. I am distressed by the levels of physical playtime children now get. The selling of school playing-fields for development and cutting PE in favour of more classroom instruction are disasters in the making. Such short-sighted policies may save money today, but at the expense of our children's health in the decades to come.

Even more harmful than decreasing exercise, however, is how food itself has changed. As we delegate more and more of our food preparation to fast-food restaurants and food manufacturers, its quality has deteriorated – not just in its taste but in its fibre and nutrient content. In a sense, food manufacturers have begun the digestion process for us. We did not appreciate until quite recently that processed foods were bad and have contributed to our epidemic of obesity. We endured hunger once; now the plenty we enjoy translates directly into the load on our dinner plates. The fact that half of all restaurant meals come in the form of fast food has only worsened things. Once, the carbs we ate were less processed than they are today. More of our bread was baked at home or in local bakeries, not factories, and was made with whole grains, not flour that had been overly processed and stripped of all fibre. Back then, convenience and speedy preparation weren't the highest ideals food aspired to – we were in less of a rush, and home cooking meant starting with raw ingredients. Rice had more of its fibre intact, and had to be cooked slowly. Potatoes weren't sliced and frozen or powdered and bought in a box. Children's after-school snacks weren't limited to what could be microwaved. More of what we ate had shelf lives measured in days, not months and sometimes years!

We didn't require large infusions of sugar in every meal, starting with our breakfast cereal and continuing at every feeding up to the late-night snack of crisps. We weren't confronted with fast-food restaurants and chocolate-chip biscuit stands and sandwich bars at every street corner.

Even the impulse towards healthy eating brought us closer to this unhealthy state. Next time you visit a supermarket, examine the nutritional information on all the 'low-fat' products: Invariably, you'll find that pro-cessed carbs have been added to replace the fats. Or notice how many breads there are labelled 'vitamin-enriched' or 'fortified', which means so much of the natural fibre (which contains the vitamins) has been stripped away that some nutrients had to be added back in!

I realize that I'm describing more than any one patient's eating patterns: It's the general attitude to nutrition that's to blame for what's happening internally to many millions of us. Usually, the serious damage doesn't show up until you're in your fifties or even sixties. But the invisible harm is being done decades earlier, setting the stage for the future catastrophe.

The cure for this, luckily, is the same as the solution to the overweight problem that vexes millions of people who aren't terribly concerned about their cardiac well-being decades from now. It's what I've tried to codify in a sensible, practical, easy to remember and follow eating plan that the rest of this book is devoted to explaining. But as far as I'm concerned, this is the true goal of any great diet. Looking good on the outside is important, I know. But having beautiful, physically fit blood vessels and healthy blood chemistry as a result makes it that much more important.

MY SOUTH BEACH DIET:

JUDY H.:

I WENT FROM A SIZE 34 TO A SIZE 20.

I 'm 55. I'm divorced. About a year or so ago, I weighed 27½ stone.

It runs in my family. On my mother's side, all the parents and their oldest child – but only the oldest child, which includes me – are heavy. I was fairly thin most of my younger years. But after I had my son and daughter, I gained weight, and I would yo-yo up and down. I've been on many diets over the years, and I've always been able to lose weight. Once I lost 7 stone on a very strict diet. But I eventually gained it back.

I was never a breakfast person. Wasn't a coffee drinker. I don't smoke, I don't drink. I would eat nothing all morning, not even a snack. And for lunch I would just eat whatever everybody else in my office was having. I didn't put a lot of thought into it. It could be Chinese food, it could be hamburgers. Whatever the girls were ordering. We had a lot of full lunches brought in – pasta was a big thing for me at lunch.

After that I didn't eat again until dinner. No snacks in the afternoon. And then dinner-time was usually meat, a vegetable, a salad, and a starch. Pasta. Or potatoes. I was never a rice person. But I really liked my other carbs – pizza and sandwiches too. I would rather eat a sandwich than sit down and have steak and potatoes. Pastry also – I love pastries. Not a sweet eater, but I liked my breads and desserts. I wasn't a big fizzy drinks fan. I was never really that thirsty – that was another problem.

Everybody said, 'Go to Weight Watchers.' 'Try Jenny Craig.' I've tried everything. One day I was talking to one of the girls in our office and I said to her, 'Hey, you look great.' And she says, 'Oh, I'm on this diet I just heard about, Dr Agatston's diet.' So she gave me a copy. And I just took it and ran with it. And I've lost 9½ stone in the year or so since.

But at first when I looked at this diet and I saw that it restricted carbs, I said, 'I'll never be able to do it.' But then I said, 'Well, you *gotta* do it.' So I decided: There will be no more bread in the house. No more milk in the house. I must have had 20 boxes of pasta in the kitchen. Threw it all out. I told my daughter, 'Look, if you need a sandwich, go buy a roll and make one. I just can't have it lying around here.' I got rid of everything, and I never brought it back into the house.

And, still, to this day, I miss my bread – I really do. I would kill to sit down and eat Italian bread with some butter. But I won't do it. Because I know I can't control myself with that stuff. In the past few weeks I found myself close to slipping a little – like wanting just a taste of this or that. Things I wouldn't even think of tasting before. I asked somebody I know at work, 'Do you notice me doing anything different?' And he said, 'Yes, I do – when we have lunch in the office, before you wouldn't touch one morsel of something that you weren't supposed to have. Now you'll take a spoon or two.' So maybe I've slipped a little. But that's good to know. I'm going to have to watch it with carbs for the rest of my life.

The first day wasn't bad. I felt, like, I *have* to do it. This is my last chance. And I started and just stayed on it. I could see the difference the first week. Within six weeks I lost 3½ stone. After that, I began to incorporate more fruits and vegetables into my diet, and some mayonnaise in my tuna, things like that. But I stayed away from having even a little bit of cereal or porridge. No starches. Now and then, as a treat, I might have allowed myself a little piece of a roll of something. But I stop myself. If I go out, I only go to restaurants where I know I can eat the food. I'm not going to kill myself and sit in an Italian restaurant. I know better. I'll go to a Chinese restaurant if I know they don't use MSG (monosodium glutamate). You can pick out your own fresh meat and vegetables and things and they'll stir-fry them for you. So I go there maybe twice a week. I'm a big seafood person. I'll eat mussels, crab legs, prawns. They have green beans cooked with oil and garlic. I'll eat a whole plate of them. Iced tea with Sweet'n Low or a diet drink. I go home full. That's my treat, twice a week.

And I don't go to any fast-food places at all any more, because there's really nothing I can have. My only big treat, once a month – I go to McDonald's and get a low-fat fruit yogurt. It has carbs in it, but I have it anyway. See, they don't tell you about the carbs. So it says 'low-fat' but there might be sugar in it. The fruit might have been frozen in sugar. They make you believe you're having something healthy, but you're not. You have to read every single ingredient before you buy anything. Like when I go to the supermarket, I buy the sugar-free lollies. When I want something sweet, I'll eat them. And if I have a bad night where I really crave something, I might eat three or four of them. But it gets me over that hump. I make sugar-free jelly. I buy diet drinks. I have one cup of coffee a day, in the morning.

Now I even try to eat breakfast. I'll have an egg and maybe two slices of bacon. Or I'll take cold meat and just roll it up with some low-fat cheese and a sliced tomato. I'm still not a big breakfast person. But I find that it gets the fire burning.

No baked goods. At work, if they bring in tuna on French bread, I might eat a little of the bread with the tuna. But the times I do that are very few and far between. I can't allow myself. Even now, I'm in a little bit of a stall. I've been yo-yo'ing with the same 10 pounds for the last three months. I was back home in Pennsylvania for three weeks, and I went to a wedding, a birthday party, and Thanksgiving – and I didn't gain anything. At my nephew's wedding I had the salmon, I ate the salad, and that was it. I didn't have any wedding cake.

On Thanksgiving my brother-in-law made me aubergine and I had salad. I didn't have the turkey and stuffing and potatoes and all that. My family's very supportive when I go home. And it felt good when I went back because I hadn't seen them for a while – at one point I lost 4 stone between visits, and the next time I saw them I had lost 2 more. By the time of my latest visit back home I had dropped about 9 stone. I was going to meet an old friend from high school for dinner, and he walked right past me. Then he turned around and said, 'Judy? You look no different than 25, 30 years ago.' I gave him the biggest kiss. I'm still heavy, don't get me wrong, but on this diet I went from a size 34 to a size 20. This is the only diet that has ever really worked for me.

chapter ten

how to eat in a restaurant

B ecause this diet is designed to be practical and user-friendly, it's easy to stick to the rules even if you dine out often.

This is not usually the case for weight-loss plans, which is why it was so important to us that the South Beach Diet work no matter who does the cooking. The dining out dilemma was especially painful for people on low-fat regimes. You either had to give the restaurant staff the third degree – What are the chicken breasts sautéed in? What exactly is in the vinaigrette? – or you had to bring your own food and hope no one objected. Even if they didn't, there was something sad about seeing healthy adults hovering over their Tupperware containers while their tablemates enjoyed fine dinners.

The overall trend in restaurant food over the past few decades has been towards healthy and fresh. Olive oil has become a staple. Every day it seems we read more about the benefits of certain fish. Menus include lots of grilled items and few that are fried. As a result, it's not hard to eat out when you're on the South Beach Diet.

Of course, you still have to watch what you're doing, but eating out is a good time to indulge in the things you love most, if only because doing so makes it a little easier to be moderate the rest of the time. There are a few strategies, many of which we've learned from patients, that can help you eat wisely even when you're on the town.

Here's a simple one: Eat something 15 minutes before you arrive at the restaurant. Just a little snack – a protein of some kind. A piece of low-fat cheese is good because you can carry it in your handbag or briefcase. It will begin the process of filling you up so that when it's time to order, you won't be feeling ravenous.

I recommend this also because it will help you get beyond the most treacherous part of any restaurant meal: the bread basket. Typically, you arrive, you're hungry, and there it is – fresh, perhaps warm and fragrant, and loaded with bad carbs. It won't really do much to satisfy your hunger, but it will jolt your bloodstream with glucose and set you up for reactive hypoglycemia and cravings for the rest of the evening.

Many people on the diet take the preemptive measure of telling the waiter to skip the bread basket altogether, which is a great idea as long as your fellow diners don't mind. If they do, you can always ask them to take their bread, *then* banish the basket.

Here's another good idea for the moment you arrive: Order soup, preferably a clear stock or consommé. The point of this, besides being filling, is that it extends your eating time. That's a good idea because there's a lag between when your belly begins to fill and when your brain notices it – maybe 20 minutes, the experts say. This fact explains why it's so easy to reach the point where you feel uncomfortably stuffed. Especially today, when speed is valued in both the preparation and the consumption of food, this is a danger. We eat so fast that we zoom right by the point of satiety and keep feeding ourselves until all of a sudden, we feel like we'll explode.

Starting a meal with stock begins the process of satisfying your hunger and initiates the signals to your brain that you are on the road to fullness. Anything that takes the edge off your hunger now is good, because it will keep you from eating more than you really need in a little while, when the food arrives.

If you peeped inside the bread basket and found a piece of the good, granary variety, you may decide to indulge yourself. If you do, dip it in olive oil, which will slow down the absorption of starches and contribute to your feeling of fullness. Believe it or not, bread with oil or even a little butter is better for your diet than bread alone, despite the fact that you're adding calories.

Here's another tip: Go to restaurants serving Mediterranean-style food. I don't just mean Italian – in fact, Italian restaurants can be dangerous because of how pasta and bread tend to dominate the meal. I'm thinking of Greek and Middle Eastern food. These are cuisines that employ lots of olive oil, which is always a plus. You can have hummus (paste made from chickpeas) on pitta bread, which is a *big* improvement over white bread and butter, and it's more flavoursome, too. You'll find good, whole grains such as tabouleh and couscous, which takes the place of potatoes or rice. And usually, these cuisines rely on spices and condiments rather than sweeteners to make the dishes taste good.

And if you *do* go Italian, try to structure the meal the way they do in Italy – in courses, with a modest serving of *al dente* pasta topped with a healthy tomato sauce, followed by a main course of meat or fish and fresh vegetables, including either leafy green ones like Batavian endive or spinach or crucifers like broccoli, plus a salad dressed in olive oil. In Italy, you don't sit down in front of a huge dish of pasta with a bottomless bread basket and call it dinner. That's why Italians can eat pasta twice a day and not suffer the obesity rates we see in the United States. In many restaurants you can request a half-portion of pasta as your appetizer. If you try this you'll see that it satisfies. It's important to eat enough good fats (the entrée and the olive oil) and good carbs (the vegetables and the salad) to counter the starches in the pasta.

We all tend to assume that restaurants serving Asian food are by definition healthy. The various Asian national diets tend to be heavy on fish and vegetables, light on heavy meats or sweets. But that's not always the case in Asian restaurants in Britain. One major difference is portion size – we are accustomed to a lot more food on our plates. And because everybody hates waste, we tend to finish what's there. Another significant difference is in the rice. Asians have always used the whole grain, meaning the fibre is there, too, and your digestive system has to work to get at the starch. In this country, and even increasingly in Asian cities, a more processed variety of white rice is used. That change substantially increases the glycemic load of a meal.

Something else you may not realize: MSG (monosodium glutamate), the flavouring agent, is made from beets, which are a healthy vegetable but have a very high glycemic index. They're loaded with sugar, in other words, though it is disguised fairly well in your average Chinese take-away dinner.

Stay away from rice or potatoes in *any* restaurant. Order a double serving of the vegetables instead. And never order anything that's fried. Roasted, grilled, braised, baked, steamed, even sautéed – all right. If there's a sauce, ask for it on the side – that doesn't mean you won't have any, but I guarantee that you'll be satisfied using half of what they would have ladled on.

As for drinks, start with water as soon as you're seated, but feel free to have a glass or two of red wine (which is actually good for your health and not terribly fattening) instead of white wine, spirits or, worst of all, beer.

For dessert, don't be too hard on yourself. If you eat out four times a week you need to say no most of the time, but if it feels like a special event, make the most of it. If fresh fruit would do the trick, have that. If fruit with ice-cream is what you need, that's fine, too. You can ask for them in separate dishes and make your own dessert, using three teaspoons of ice-cream topped by the fresh fruit. If only the most decadent chocolate cake will suffice, go ahead and order it – along with enough forks for everyone at the table. Have three bites only and eat them as slowly as possible. Then send the rest away with the first passing waiter. Try this experiment at home: Have three bites of any dessert, then stop and put the rest aside for a few minutes. You'll see that it was as satisfying as if you had eaten the whole thing. And you'll still respect yourself in the morning.

Of course, all this presupposes that you're eating in a normal, sit-down restaurant. But the fact is that most American dining out these days is done in fast-food places. It's hard to think of any strategy that might actually help there. Everything seems to conspire to deliver the worst meal possible, at least from our perspective.

Start by eliminating all the main attractions. No burgers (too many saturated fats in the meat and the cooking oil, too many carbs in the bun). No fish, either, since the coating and the cooking method make it even more fattening than the burger. No chips (the worst part of the meal from the glycemic index point of view, both the potatoes and the ketchup). No fizzy drink, which leads to pure sugar rush. Look at how fast-food restaurants emphasize their worse fare – even the offer to 'supersize' is simply a way to sell you excessive amounts of the cheapest part of the meal, the drink and the chips. The emphasis in fast food is on big, sweet, fat, and *fast* – everything that has made obesity such a problem in America today.

If you can visit a fast-food restaurant and limit yourself to salad (with oil and vinegar instead of any other dressing) and plain grilled chicken breast (in the places that serve it), accompanied by water or coffee, you can do all right. Chicken nuggets or fried chicken are bad news – like the fish, they consist of a lot of deep-fried bread over a little meat, which has been cooked in a trans fatty substance. Otherwise, you can't really eat at these places and follow any sort of healthful diet. That's no surprise, is it?'

MY SOUTH BEACH DIET

JUDITH W.:

I WENT DOWN THREE DRESS SIZES, AND MY CHOLESTEROL IS DOWN, TOO.

I've had high blood pressure and angina for many years, and heart trouble runs in my family. I had a triple bypass in 1990, and I was the baby in the cardiac ward. My mother had already had one, and my sister had one, too. A few years ago I needed a new cardiologist and I went to Dr Agatston. The first thing he told me was that I had to lose weight, and since I weighed 12 stone at that time I knew he was right. He didn't tell me anything I didn't know. But he gave me the inspiration and he suggested this diet.

I cut out all of the carbs that I was supposed to cut out, and the sugar, too. They told me not to buy no-fat, because that just meant the foods were higher in sugars. But I did buy 2 percent milk and low-fat cheeses. Before I went on the diet, I never ate breakfast. But I would snack in the evening. I never snacked on sweets; it was always fruit or pretzels. I always ate baked potatoes, but never with butter, because I thought potatoes were all right. I'd have chips whenever I wanted. Of course I had a roll with my hamburger. I was trying to eat sensibly, but I wasn't really killing myself at it. And slowly but surely, I gained a lot of weight. I was in a panic when I started the diet, because I had never looked that big in my life. Never.

Once I got through the strict phase I began adding back some carbs. But not many. I don't trust carbs. I'll eat wholemeal pasta, but just a small amount. Brown rice, too. That's about it. Cheerios. No potatoes at all – only sweet potatoes. I bake them. I won't eat a whole potato, though – half. Sugar-free jams or jellies, if necessary, but I don't have a sweet tooth, so I'm lucky. When I added the carbs back, I still kept losing weight. I will now, occasionally, have a sandwich made with stone-ground wholemeal bread – thin-sliced, if I can get it.

I lost 2 stone over the course of maybe six months, and three years later I've kept it all off. I went down three dress sizes, and my cholesterol is down, too. My husband said it's the most expensive diet I ever went on, because I had to throw out all my clothes and start over. I'm an attorney, so I have a very expensive business wardrobe. And we go to a lot of evening functions, too. I love it – I finally have a great excuse for a whole new wardrobe.

chapter eleven

back to cardiology

As I've noted, I came to study diet and weight loss only via my speciality of preventive cardiology. I fully agree with a quote from the famous Framingham Heart Study group: 'A heart attack or stroke should indicate a failure of medical therapy rather than the beginning of medical intervention.' I am convinced that preventing most heart attacks and strokes is not a pipe-dream but something that is feasible today. Even people who come to me with family histories of premature heart disease can, in most cases, overcome the genetic predisposition. The important thing is to begin prevention early. The earlier it is started, the easier it is to prevent future catastrophe. In too many cases, the first manifestation of heart attack or stroke is also the last.

Diet is, of course, a crucial component of our prevention strategy. For many patients, particularly those with diabetes or prediabetes, it is our primary focus. Exercise is important, but proper diet is absolutely the most essential element.

If you neglect that, you may someday have to take your chances with the so-called miracles of modern cardiology – angioplasty, coronary artery bypass, transplant, perhaps even the totally artificial heart. Such measures may restore sufficient cardiac function to keep you alive. These are the extreme, invasive, last-ditch efforts required once the patient and his or her doctors have proven unable to keep the cardiovascular system working as nature intended. In some cases there's a disease or dysfunction that caused the ailment. But overwhelmingly, most problems cardiologists treat can be *prevented*.

Exercise

As with diet, the goal here should be to find an exercise plan that will seem less like an intervention and more like part of your existing lifestyle — something you can incorporate easily into your routine. You can seek the greatest cardiac workout ever, one that will put you in marathoner shape. But if it requires you to remake your life it will probably be a flop. You'll never maintain it over the long haul, and the discouragement alone will leave you worse off than before you started.

Besides, you don't really *need* a Marine Corps-level exercise programme to have a healthy heart. What you need is a daily dose of activity that will achieve the desired effect as efficiently as possible. Anything beyond that is optional. Too many people approach this as an all-or-nothing proposition — they start out with a high-intensity programme, keep it up for a short spell, tire of it, and go back to doing nothing at all. Better to find a 30-minute workout you'll do daily. You won't burn a lot of calories each session, but the cumulative effect will be beneficial in every way. At the very least you'll offset the pound or two that most middle-aged people put on per year without even noticing. Clearly, people who exercise often and with gusto are better off than those who don't. It's not just a matter of cardiac health, either: Moving your body and pushing its limits puts you in a healthy frame of mind, I believe, in addition to the many other benefits.

The first thing you need is some kind of aerobic workout. You don't have to spend an hour on the treadmill, stair machine, elliptical trainer, or running track, however. Here's what I recommend: A brisk 20-minute walk every day. Don't run unless you really want to. Live by this easy-to-remember rule: As soon as you begin to perspire, you can call it quits. You get the majority of benefit from exercise during the first 20 minutes or so. If you want to stop at that point, it's all right. You've achieved your purpose. But you have to do it for 20 minutes, vigorously and religiously, every day. If you like swimming and it's possible to do it year round, be my guest. Again, you don't need to train like an Olympic hopeful. Twenty minutes.

In addition to that, I recommend some stretching, mainly because it ensures that you won't hurt yourself doing whatever other exercise you choose. But stretching is also good for circulation and lung function, which improves everything else. And it keeps your blood vessels young and healthy.

Finally, you need to do some weight training. It will improve your muscle–fat ratio, which will in turn raise your metabolism, causing your body to burn fuel faster even when you're asleep. You don't have to become a bodybuilder, but increasing lean body mass – meaning anything other than fat – is important. For women especially, weight training is good for how it builds bone density, which will forestall the effects of osteoporosis as you age.

In addition to all that, exercise lowers your blood pressure and bad cholesterol. Exercise regularly and eat properly, and you're doing just about all you can to ensure a healthy cardiac future. You're already doing far more for yourself than medical science can do for you.

Before a sustained workout (longer than 90 minutes), it may help to eat some low-glycemic carb, such as low-fat yogurt, porridge, or pumpernickel bread. Eat it at least two hours before exercising so you'll have a good supply of carbohydrates to give you an energy boost. After exercise you need to replenish glycogen fuel stores. You can even allow yourself white bread or potatoes at this time.

Medications and supplements

Earlier in the book, I described my journey as a cardiologist firmly committed to the 'prevention first' approach, especially as it pertains to diet. But nutrition and exercise alone can't always ensure cardiac health. In the late 1980s a new class of amazing cholesterol-lowering drugs known as the statins – medications such as Lescol, Zocor, and Lipitor – became available. With these, we were able to cut cholesterol quite easily and dramatically – 20 to 30 percent initially, and now, up to 50 percent. By taking these drugs, we thought, patients could have their cake and eat it, too – literally. They could diet or not and still enjoy low cholesterol. Of course, statins did nothing for the waistline. Still, the prevailing wisdom was to forget about diet and take the drugs. Statins were (and still are) expensive, and there is no research into the long-term effects of taking them. However, studies showed that the incidence of heart attacks could be diminished by approximately 30 percent with this class of medication.

I won't burden you with the scientific explanation behind statins. These compounds work by blocking the production of cholesterol in the liver. There has been some controversy associated with them, mainly over the possibility that they cause liver problems. One statin drug, Benecor, was withdrawn from the market after some patients taking it died of liver failure. There is no known problem with the statin drugs now on the market, however, despite the occasional scare that arises in the papers or on TV news shows. The benefits of statins far outweigh the potential hazards. Among physicians, there has never been any serious doubt about the wisdom of taking them. Consider this: Most cardiologists I know over the age of 40 are taking a statin drug, even doctors with no sign or history of heart trouble. The medication isn't cheap but the results are worth it.

Supplements, too, have become a big part of cardiac care in recent years.

Most people know to take an aspirin every day to thin the blood slightly and help prevent heart attack and strokes. It's worth emphasizing here what a blessing aspirin really is when it comes to cardiac prevention – it's so common and inexpensive that some people forget it's an important part of any heart-healthy regime.

For years we've been hearing how the classic antioxidant vitamins (A, C, and E) would help prevent heart attack, stroke, and cancer. Recently, though, multiple studies have failed to support these hopes with science. The good news is that vitamins and supplements don't do any harm (except to your wallet). The bad news is that they also appear to do no good. There's some evidence that the natural form of vitamin E, called d alpha tocopherol, is effective in preventing heart attacks and strokes. But further study is needed. My advice is to boost your body's supply of antioxidants by exercising and eating fruits and vegetables, which are rich in nutrients. I hedge my bet by suggesting a single daily multivitamin.

The news about taking fish-oil supplements, in capsule form, continues to be good, however. Just as we advise people to eat plenty of fish high in beneficial omega-3 oils, such as salmon and tuna, we suggest these capsules. They lower triglycerides and make the blood cells less sticky. They've also been found to prevent sudden death due to cardiac arrhythmia – the sudden, potentially fatal stoppage of the normal heartbeat. (For more on the marvels of fish oil, read Dr Andrew L. Stoll's excellent book, *The Omega-3 Connection*.)

I, personally, take one aspirin, two fish oil capsules, a statin drug, and an angiotensin-converting enzyme inhibitor, commonly known as an ACE inhibitor, which prevents inflammation, daily.

Recently, a study turned up another potentially important addition to the list of supplements. Some men undergo a kind of menopause equivalent associated with the normal drop in their testosterone levels starting in their fifties. We've always known that this hormone fuels sex drive. Now we find that it may also have something to do with cardiac function. Studies now indicate that men who have heart attacks often are found to have lower-than-normal testosterone levels. Diabetic men, too, tend to have low testosterone. Injections of this hormone in men who make no change in diet still results in lessened central obesity – it now seems as though the drop in testosterone may be another reason men gain weight as they age.

We never knew any of this before because we measured testosterone only in men with sexual dysfunction. Now we see the impact this hormone has on the entire obesity–cardiac health connection. I test for it in all my male patients and prescribe a testosterone gel (which is rubbed on the skin) for those whose levels are low.

Advanced blood testing

Lowering total cholesterol is an important goal in preventive care, but it's not nearly enough. In fact, most people who suffer heart attacks have average cholesterol levels. The fact is that one person can have a low cholesterol number and be at grave risk of a heart attack, while someone else with a higher figure will be fine. The familiar total cholesterol figure *alone* doesn't tell the entire story.

By now, most people will realize there are two basic types of cholesterol – the so-called good kind (high-density lipoproteins, or HDLs) and the bad (low-density, or LDLs). The ratio of good to bad is an important factor, one which is today commonly measured by diagnostic blood work.

But there are also other factors that must be considered, and for this reason advanced lipid testing has now become a requirement in any serious cardiac care.

The most sophisticated blood labs are now capable of measuring five different subgroups of HDL and seven of LDL. One thing they evaluate is the *size* of the cholesterol particles. In essence, large particles are good and small ones are bad. Large HDLs have proved to be more efficient at their job of clearing away bad fats than small HDLs are. Even more important, though, is the difference between large and small LDL particles.

The small ones squeeze more easily under the lining of blood vessels, where they form the plaque that narrows arteries. Larger LDL particles can't slide beneath the linings so well, and as a result their potential for harm is smaller.

Advanced blood lipid testing has been pioneered by the Lawrence Berkeley National Laboratory of the University of California at Berkeley and its commercial arm, the Berkeley HeartLab. Dr Robert Superko, medical director of the lab, has done an outstanding job of educating doctors in the use of advanced blood testing for treating patients. When the cholesterol sub-classes are taken along with other advanced tests, including Lp(a), homocysteine, and others, we can explain over 90 percent of the heart disease we see. We can also test for high sensitivity to C-reactive protein – CRP – a marker for inflammation of the blood vessel lining. Dr Paul Ridker, of Harvard, did the groundbreaking research proving that inflammation of the arteries can play a big role in arteriosclerosis and heart attacks. Measuring this inflammation can predict who is a candidate for a heart attack, even in patients with normal or low cholesterol. It's interesting to note that people with prediabetes or diabetes often have normal cholesterols but high CRPs.

EBT scanning

There's a final medical measure that must be taken to promote heart health, one with which I am extremely familiar: the use of electron beam tomography (EBT) as a non-invasive tool for examining the heart while it does its job. More than the electrocardiograph (ECG) or even the CT scan, this technology has the power to tell us the exact condition of the organ itself and the blood vessels that serve it. We can obtain critical information using this that no other diagnostic tests provide.

In June of 1988, I worked with my colleagues Warren Janowitz, David King, and Manuel Viamonte to come up with a method of identifying cardiac plaque simply, accurately, and painlessly, without having to invade the body. We used a then-revolutionary type of CT scan called electron beam tomography, or EBT.

This fast (5 minutes), painless (no needles or dye, no undressing) CT scanner was developed by a brilliant physicist, Douglas Boyd. The procedure takes pictures in a fraction of a second, freezing the image of the beating heart. With a conventional CT scanner the beating heart shows up as a blur. With General Electric's EBT, high resolution of the coronary arteries can be obtained, allowing us to see and measure calcium deposits, which are accurate indicators of the total amount of arteriosclerosis inside the vessel walls. Using these images we can identify who needs to be treated in advance of a heart attack or stroke. By treating the patient with diet, exercise, and medication, we can retest and monitor the effectiveness of the treatment.

Proper diet and exercise are still the most important things you can do to take care of your heart. Combine those with advanced lipid testing, aggressive lipid controls (statins and supplements), and the EBT, and the vast majority of heart attacks and even strokes can be averted.

MY SOUTH BEACH DIET

NANCY A.:

I DIDN'T GAIN ANYTHING DURING PREGNANCY.

I was working at Mount Sinai Hospital, in the child-care centre, where some of the children's parents work in the cardiovascular department. They invited us to be part of some research they were doing, and in exchange we'd get free diet consultations for three months. We had to pick a diet at random, and I ended up with the modified carbohydrate diet, which later became known as the South Beach Diet.

When I started I weighed 12 stone. For the previous five years, I had tried everything to lose weight. I tried appetite suppressant drugs three separate times. That's how I gained so much weight – I gained everything back double every time I stopped. I tried Slim-Fast, too. After a while I was getting really hungry from just drinking shakes, and so I went back to my regular eating habits. On my own, I decided to do salads only. That didn't work, either – I didn't have enough willpower. I would get even hungrier after eating a salad.

I'm Spanish, so we were raised on Spanish foods, which tend to have a lot of fat. I had to cut down on that stuff, fried foods especially. But every time I went a month or two eating healthy foods, I would crave my traditional dishes. Pork in the oven with rice, fried plantains, fried chicken. I couldn't stop myself from wanting it. I'm also a sweets person, so cheesecake here and there, a biscuit here and there. I work in a child-care centre, so we have tons of snacks for the children. After a big dinner, I would eat a bowl of ice-cream, or cereal, or cake.

The first two weeks on the South Beach Diet were the toughest – just low-fat meats and vegetables and water. Around the second week, I was going crazy. It was psychologically stressful. But I did it. Going to visit the nutritionist was helpful. Within those first weeks I think I cheated once, on cheesecake. A couple of times I was tempted to have rice, but I had stopped buying it, so there was none in the house. It kind of killed me, not having it around.

After the two strict weeks were up, it got a lot easier. I was able to have more variety. I went to the store and went crazy buying everything that was on the list. I was able to have fruit. And vegetables – I even started eating ones I'd never tried before. I was so eager to have more variety. Broccoli. Asparagus. Anything I saw.

After the three-month period, I had got down from around 12 to 10 stone. Actually, on the day I made the final visit to the nutritionist, I found out that I was pregnant. And I had been trying for five years. In fact, I had given up trying. And here I was, pregnant at last. I don't actually know what triggered that, but I think it's because I had been so overweight and not eating right. Something must have changed. And I had a perfect pregnancy.

I kept the weight off for two years. I didn't gain anything during the pregnancy. And only recently did I start to slide backwards. I've been neglecting myself a little, and some of the weight is back on. When you have a three-year-old and you're working at a day-care centre, you're surrounded by sweets. But I just got another copy of the diet from the nutritionist, and I'm going back again.

chapter twelve

why do people fail on the South Beach Diet?

I t's a good question, because occasionally some *do* fail. We're always looking at the reasons, trying to find ways to improve the programme. Most people who go on it report that taking the plunge is surprisingly easy. That's partly because the South Beach Diet doesn't require you to give up everything you love. We strongly encourage you to eat until you're no longer hungry, and to snack when you feel the need, even during the stringent first two weeks.

But we recognize that it's also easy at the start because it's human nature to be gung-ho at the beginning of *any* new health regime. You're feeling motivated, and so you're optimistic and full of resolve and determination to get your life and your looks back on track. Before you know it you're watching the pounds begin to melt away. You see the numbers on your scale descend, and you dig out garments that were once uncomfortably snug – or maybe even impossibly tight – and suddenly they begin to seem possible again. Sticking with the programme is easy with so much good stuff going on.

Then what happens?

To a degree, failure comes because of the programme's success. People lose anywhere from 8 to 13 pounds during the first two weeks. At that point you switch from the strictest phase to Phase 2. This is when you begin reintroducing some of the carbs you cut completely in Phase 1. The purpose of adding them back, as I've said, is manifold: Some carbs are good for you, and we want you to be on a healthy diet that's as close to 'normal' eating as possible. That means you're going to eat fruit, and bread or pasta once in a while, and even a dessert here and there.

You continue losing weight in Phase 2, but not at the same speed as you did in Phase 1. Depending on how much you want to lose, it may take up to a year or even longer.

For some dieters, that's a disappointment. And they remember that Phase 1 wasn't so restrictive. They couldn't eat certain things they love, but they never went hungry or felt discomfort. So they decide to stay on Phase 1 indefinitely, until they reach their goal.

Now, I know plenty of dieters who have made that decision and succeeded. But I know plenty more who have failed.

Here's why they fail: Phase 1 isn't meant to be a long-term eating plan. You're limited to a fairly small palette of foods – grilled lean meats and fish, vegetables, low-fat cheeses and salads, all either steamed or prepared using good fats such as olive oil and rapeseed oil. For snacks, nuts and chunks of low-fat cheddar, and that's about it.

From a culinary point of view, it's a perfectly acceptable diet – for two or three weeks.

After that, it gets a little dull. That, we find, is where the trouble starts.

That's when dieters begin to improvise, only they do so improperly. They mix in their bad old habits – just once in a while, mind you. They follow Phase 1 but they add in a handful of bourbon biscuits every night. Even that's not exactly it: They add in one biscuit after dinner, realize it tasted pretty good and probably did no harm, and then increase it to three every night. Three biscuits a night with no noticeable harm makes it easy to allow a small bag of corn chips at 4 o'clock one afternoon. If you're doing all right with three biscuits and corn chips, it doesn't seem so unwise to indulge a craving for pizza and beer on the weekend.

Before long, you're cheating more than dieting.

When you realize how badly you've strayed, you may do what lots of our people have tried: You'll revert at once to the strict Phase 1 plan. But when you do, it seems even more monotonous than it did the first time.

At that point, you may just surrender. Some people do. If you're lucky, you won't end up weighing more than you did before you started the diet, though backsliding has a way of sending you to a point even beyond where you began.

It's a diet truism that you can't lose in a day what took you years to put on. We all accept that, and yet it's hard not to try the quick fix. Sometimes the end result is weight gain, not loss.

It's important for people to like the food they eat. Eating is meant to bring pleasure, even when you're trying to lose weight. That's a sensible way to think about food, and it's one of the basic principles of the South Beach Diet. Which is why we strongly urge all the people we counsel to switch to Phase 2 after the second week, no matter how tempting it is to remain on Phase 1. This is a long-term diet, and the three-phase approach is an important part of its success. It may take longer to lose the weight this way. But your chances of losing it and keeping it off are better.

Daily challenges

A second reason for failure has more to do with how everyday life intrudes on our plans. You've reached your target weight. Now you're in Phase 3, the diet's maintenance stage, meaning you still have to eat a certain way to *keep* the weight off. This, if you stick with the programme, is how you'll eat for the rest of your life.

What kind of intrusions am I talking about? People who travel a good deal, especially on business, are at a high risk of diet failure. Travel is disruption, especially of your normal eating routines. That's dangerous. It's especially so nowadays when in-flight food service has become a thing of the past. Once, you could plan ahead and order the special vegetarian or kosher meal and you'd get something fresh and healthy and made to order. You could easily bypass the meat with gravy, mashed potatoes, peas and carrots, applesauce, and fruit cobbler for dessert.

Today, more than likely all you've been served is some tropical mix or honey-roasted peanuts with a beer or fizzy drink. Except for the nuts, it's all carbs and sugars.

By the time you've landed and made it to your hotel, it's way past your meal-time. With the change in time zones, it may even be past your bed-time. But you're wired up from the trip, and famished. The first thing you do is pick up the room service menu and overorder – maybe a Caesar salad with roast chicken breast would be enough to satisfy your hunger, but you hear yourself requesting the turkey club sandwich with chips and a milk shake. You regret the decision as soon as you hang up the phone, but when the food arrives you somehow manage to force it all down, along with a beer from the minibar to make you drowsy enough to sleep.

Next day you eat properly but as you near your normal dinner-time you're stuck in a working session at the home office, and it's not until 7.30 – when you're starving once again – that somebody thinks to order in a few pizzas and soft drinks. And so you end another day loaded with bad carbs.

Long working days, whether at home or on the road, are a main culprit in diet failure. It's the disruption of normal meal-times that leads you to overeat when the food finally arrives. Or you're one of those modern-day road warriors, a businessperson or sales rep who spends hours in a car, which makes it easy to grab an unhealthy lunch or snack at a fast-food counter and wolf it down in the car park.

Sometimes it's the work-related stress that makes it easy to fall back into comforting old habits. People who eat when they feel psychological or emotional pressure tend to fall off the diet wagon. Think of the items we call comfort foods – invariably it's either baked goodies, like cakes and pies and chocolate chip biscuits, or dishes such as macaroni cheese.

I can't tell you how many people went off the diet in the fall and winter of 2001. The terrorist attacks jarred us out of our sense of safety, or they made weight seem like an awfully trivial concern in the larger scheme of things. That's the kind of anxiety and insecurity that seeks comfort in a sweet mouthful or a brimming dinner plate. It's hard to advise people how to cope with that kind of stress while sticking to a diet.

Elsewhere in this book I've included testimonials from people who have gone on the South Beach Diet, got down to their desired weight, and remained there. Here I'm going to quote someone who went on the diet, lost weight, and then backslid – so much so that today he weighs pretty much what he did when he started. His story is a good example of how, sometimes, just a momentary break in the diet can spell disaster. In its way this should be as instructive as the others. To protect the guilty, though, I won't name this dieter.

I had had an early heart attack – I'm in my fifties – and was in cardiac rehab when I finally decided it was time to lose weight. I was up around 17 stone at the time. I went to the nutritionist, and she set me up on a four-week version of the South Beach Diet.

In the first two weeks I lost about 8 pounds. But it left me feeling a little weak. Then I started adding back some carbs, and I felt better, and the weight kept coming off. Bread was my big weakness back then. I ate it with every meal, and sometimes I ate it between meals. If I went to a restaurant I'd feast on the bread basket, to the point where I wouldn't be hungry when dinner came. I'd have to take it home many times. So I cut the bread out completely.

My other big weakness was sweet things. I love biscuits, especially oatmeal raisin. I'd eat them all day long – I'd buy them fresh baked and take them into work for everyone, but I'd grab a handful every time I walked by the kitchen.

I had always eaten a lot of potatoes, too, and I had to give them up, but it wasn't too hard. Bread and biscuits were the tough ones. Waffles, too, with syrup, for breakfast. Or a Danish pastry. After I went on the diet, I cut out all the baked goods from my breakfast and just stuck with eggs. Lots of water to drink, that and decaf.

Instead of biscuits between meals, I'd have nuts. Maybe some peanuts in the middle of the afternoon. And no more dessert at night. Before I'd have more biscuits, or maybe a big bowl of cereal with milk. On the diet I had almonds for my dessert, while I was watching TV. I'd count 15 of them out of the jar like I was told, and I'd eat them slowly, one by one, so they'd last.

On Phase 2, I lost another 2 stone. And it was getting easier. At restaurants I'd ask them to take the bread away. I'd stick with meat and vegetables and felt just fine.

Then, the way you're supposed to, I started adding some carbs back to my diet. I'd have a slice of bread every couple days, for instance, or instead of bread I'd have a serving of rice. I kept losing weight, and I stayed with the diet for a whole year.

That's about when we had a big family outing to attend. A huge party. I had been good for so long that I said to myself I was going to eat anything and everything I wanted. I told myself that it would just be for one day, and that tomorrow I'd go back on the programme.

But tomorrow never came. I liked eating everything so much I didn't want to stop. In the past, if I added too many carbs and stopped losing weight, I'd just shift back on Phase 1 and take it off. This time I couldn't bring myself to do it. Before I knew it, all the weight I had lost – almost 3½ stone – was back. Now I'm planning to go back to Phase 1 again, but it'll be starting all over. This is a very good diet, and it really works. But you still have to actually *follow* it.

It's true that this particular dieter could easily have indulged his sweet tooth all day long at the family picnic, and then next morning gone back on the diet. That's how plenty of people operate: They'll give in to temptation on special occasions – a wedding, say, or on vacation, or at a fancy dinner – and then make up for it the next day. On this diet you can fall off the wagon, find that you've put on a pound or two, and easily backtrack to Phase I until you lose what you've gained.

All this makes perfect sense, of course – even to the people who fall off the wagon so hard that they undo weeks and even months of good work. It's okay to fall off once in a while, as long as you remember to get right back on!

MY SOUTH BEACH DIET

STEVE L.:

IF YOU FALL OFF THE WAGON OCCASIONALLY, YOU HOP BACK ON.

I had begun seeing Dr Agatston as my cardiologist when we moved to Florida. My first appointment with him was in his office – not in an exam room – where he pulled out his laptop and went through a little PowerPoint presentation and said, 'If we decide to work together, this is what our cardiac disease prevention protocol is like. And if you have a heart attack, then I've failed.'

Bad hearts run in my family, so it was important to me to get this under control. I've always been an athletic guy. I'm a fairly big guy, a little over six-two. And when I started this I was probably about 19 stone – which was my heaviest. I can hide it fairly well, and I can move comfortably with the weight, but it wasn't too healthy. And I'm from Minnesota – it's a meat-and-potatoes and high-carb lifestyle.

My huge weakness is bread and pasta. We moved down here from Seattle, where we had a pizza oven in our kitchen. So all my cravings were about carbs. Not sweets. But everything else. If we went to a restaurant, I could easily handle the bread basket by myself. I'd have bread a minimum of three times a day. And while I'm not a dessert guy, there would always be biscuits around.

Part of the problem also was a fair amount of ignorance on my part. I grew up under the impression that all fruits were healthy. Then I learned that some are high in sugar and some aren't. I didn't realize, for instance, that watermelon is full of sugar, whereas cantaloupe is not. Eggs, on the other hand, have moved into the positive category. I'm not a big drinker but I used to drink beer. I haven't had a beer for two-plus years.

My wife and I love to cook – and we love to eat. But we started having brown rice instead of white and sweet potatoes instead of regular ones. Root vegetables, frankly, weren't that difficult for me to give up. We've discovered some really great recipes, and we grill like crazy. A lot of grilled vegetables. And much more fish than we used to eat. Bread only in limited quantities. I'll have half a bagel for breakfast. If I decide to have a sandwich for lunch, it's with either rye or pumpernickel, and it's less bread and more meat than before.

I'd gone on diets my whole life, and usually at the outset I got the heebie-jeebies, and lightheadedness, all that stuff. On this I felt absolutely fine. No side effects. I stopped caffeine for two weeks, too, and I'm a coffee hog. My wife had an enormously difficult time the first two weeks. But for me it was nothing. And we were strict. I mean, I would go to work with some pistachios and a chunk of low-fat cheese for the afternoon snack.

The huge, traumatic thing for me was bread. In the last three years we've been to Italy twice. And what we would do there is order one serving of pasta and split it between the two of us, and then we'd order some legal dishes.

In the six months I've been on the diet, I've lost about 3½ stone. I put some of that back on due to stress eating lately, but I know I can go back on the strict phase and lose it again. And with Dr Agatston's blessing, if there's something we feel an urgent craving for, we just have it. If you fall off the wagon occasionally, you hop back on. So if we go out to dinner we'll order dessert once in a while – maybe one time out of three. But just one dessert for the two of us, and we'll take a bite or two each and then send it away. Just enough to end the meal on a sweet taste. And I drink red wine only – no other alcohol. Not only have I lost the weight, but all my numbers are improved. My triglycerides, for example, went from 256 to 62 after six weeks. And that was all diet. Cholesterol numbers continue to move down.

part two

Meal Plans and Recipes

chapter thirteen

phase 1 meal plan

This, as you know by now, is the strictest phase of the diet. It's meant to last for two weeks only – just long enough to resolve the insulin resistance that was brought about by eating too many bad (mostly processed) carbs. Phase I does not have to be low carb if you eat the right carbs. It is designed to allow ample portions of protein, good fats, and the lowest-glycemic index carbs needed for satisfaction and blood sugar control. These include the low-glycemic index vegetables, which also contribute fibre, important nutrients such as heart-healthy folic acid, and other vitamins and minerals. Many salads and vegetables are unlimited. You will also have your choice of proteins from a variety of sources.

By the time this phase ends, your unhealthy cravings, especially for sweets, baked goods, and starches, will also essentially have vanished. Even though this is the strict phase, you'll notice that each day includes six different occasions to eat – three meals, snacks in mid-morning and mid-afternoon, and dessert after dinner. So you should never feel hungry, and if you do, it's possible that you're being too stingy with your portions. The South Beach Diet doesn't require you to measure what you eat in ounces, calories, or anything else – the meals should be of normal size, enough to satisfy your hunger but no more than that.

DAY ONE

Breakfast

- 150ml (6 fl oz) vegetable juice cocktail
- 2 Vegetable Quiche Cups To Go (page 125)
- Decaffeinated coffee or decaffeinated tea with skimmed milk and sugar substitute

Mid-morning snack

- 1 chunk low-fat cheese

Lunch

- Sliced grilled chicken breast on lettuce
- 2 tablespoons Balsamic Vinaigrette (page 137) or low-sugar prepared dressing
- Sugar-free jelly

Mid-afternoon snack

- Celery stuffed with 1 wedge Laughing Cow Light Cheese

Dinner

- Grilled Salmon with Rosemary (page 150)
- Steamed asparagus
- Tossed salad (mixed leaves, cucumbers, green peppers, cherry tomatoes)
- Olive oil and vinegar to taste or 2 tablespoons low-sugar prepared dressing

Dessert

- Vanilla Ricotta Crème (page 165)

DAY TWO

Breakfast

- 175ml (6 fl oz) tomato juice
- 1 egg
- 2 slices lean bacon
- Decaffeinated coffee or decaffeinated tea with skimmed milk and sugar substitute

Mid-morning snack

- 1–2 Turkey Roll-Ups (page 163)
- 2 tablespoons Coriander Mayonnaise (optional) (page 163)

Lunch

- South Beach Chopped Salad with Tuna (page 130)
- Sugar-free jelly

Mid-afternoon snack

- Celery stuffed with 1 wedge Laughing Cow Light Cheese

Dinner

- Baked chicken breast
- Roasted Aubergine and Peppers (page 156)
- Tossed salad (mixed leaves, cucumbers, green peppers, cherry tomatoes)
- 2 tablespoons Balsamic Vinaigrette (page 137) or low-sugar prepared dressing

Dessert

- Mocha Ricotta Crème (page 165)

DAY THREE

Breakfast

- 150ml (6 fl oz) vegetable juice cocktail
- Easy Asparagus and Mushroom Omelette (page 123)
- Decaffeinated coffee or decaffeinated tea with skimmed milk and sugar substitute

Mid-morning snack

- 1 chunk low-fat cheese

Lunch

- Dilled Prawn Salad with Herb-Dill Dressing (page 132)
- Sugar-free jelly

Mid-afternoon snack

- 1–2 Ham Roll-ups (page 163)
- 2 tablespoons Coriander Mayonnaise (optional) (page 163)

Dinner

- Grilled sirloin steak
- Steamed broccoli
- Grilled Tomatoes (page 159)
- Surprise South Beach Mashed 'Potatoes' (page 158)

Dessert

- Almond Ricotta Crème (page 164)

DAY FOUR

Breakfast

- 175ml (6 fl oz) tomato juice
- Eggs Florentine (1 poached egg served on 100g (4 oz) spinach sautéed in olive oil)
- 2 slices lean bacon
- Decaffeinated coffee or decaffeinated tea with skimmed milk and sugar substitute

Mid-morning snack

- Celery stuffed with 1 wedge Laughing Cow Light Cheese

Lunch

- Chef's salad (at least 25g (1 oz) each ham, turkey, and low-fat cheese on mixed leaves)
- Olive oil and vinegar to taste or 2 tablespoons low-sugar prepared dressing

Mid-afternoon snack

- Up to 10 cherry tomatoes stuffed with 100g (4 oz) low-fat cottage cheese

Dinner

- White Fish in Spring Onion and Ginger Sauce (page 151)
- Steamed mange-tout
- Shredded cabbage sautéed in olive oil

Dessert

- Mocha Ricotta Crème (page 165)

DAY FIVE

Breakfast

- 150ml (6 fl oz) vegetable juice cocktail
- Western Egg White Omelette (page 124)
- Decaffeinated coffee or decaffeinated tea with skimmed milk and sugar substitute

Mid-morning snack

- 1–2 Turkey Roll-ups (page 163)
- 2 tablespoons Coriander Mayonnaise (optional) (page 163)

Lunch

- Gazpacho (page 138)
- Grilled sirloin hamburger steak (no bun)
- Tossed salad (mixed leaves, cucumber, green peppers, cherry tomatoes)
- Olive oil and vinegar to taste or 2 tablespoons low-sugar prepared dressing

Mid-afternoon snack

- Cucumber rounds with salmon spread

Dinner

- Balsamic Chicken (page 140)
- Stewed Tomatoes and Onions (page 158)
- Steamed spinach
- Tossed salad (mixed leaves, cucumber, green peppers, cherry tomatoes)
- Olive oil and vinegar to taste or 2 tablespoons low-sugar prepared dressing

Dessert

- Almond Ricotta Crème (page 164)

DAY SIX

Breakfast

- 150ml (6 fl oz) tomato juice
- Scrambled eggs with fresh herbs and mushrooms
- 2 slices lean bacon
- Decaffeinated coffee or decaffeinated tea with skimmed milk and sugar substitute

Mid-morning snack

- 1 chunk low-fat cheese

Lunch

- Chicken Caesar salad (no croutons)
- 2 tablespoons prepared Caesar dressing

Mid-afternoon snack

- 100g (4 oz) low-fat cottage cheese with 50g (2 oz) chopped tomatoes and cucumber

Dinner

- Mahi mahi or swordfish
- Oven-roasted Vegetables (page 155)
- Rocket salad
- 2 tablespoons Balsamic Vinaigrette (page 137) or low-sugar prepared dressing

Dessert

- Lemon Zest Ricotta Crème (page 164)

DAY SEVEN

Breakfast

- 150ml (6 fl oz) vegetable juice cocktail
- Smoked Salmon Frittata (page 122)
- Decaffeinated coffee or decaffeinated tea with skimmed milk and sugar substitute

Mid-morning snack

- Celery stuffed with 1 wedge Laughing Cow Light Cheese

Lunch

- Crab Cobb Salad (page 133)
- Sugar-free jelly

Mid-afternoon snack

- 2 slices low-fat (light) mozzarella cheese with 2 slices fresh tomato sprinkled with balsamic vinegar, olive oil, and freshly ground black pepper

Dinner

- Marinated London Broil (page 146)
- Spinach-stuffed Mushrooms (page 157)
- Surprise South Beach Mashed 'Potatoes' (page 158)
- Tossed salad (mixed leaves, cucumber, green peppers, cherry tomatoes)
- Olive oil and vinegar to taste or 2 tablespoons low-sugar prepared dressing

Dessert

- Lime Zest Ricotta Crème (page 166)

DAY EIGHT

Breakfast

- Light Spinach Frittata with Tomato Salsa (page 121)
- Decaffeinated coffee or decaffeinated tea with skimmed milk and sugar substitute

Mid-morning snack

- 1 chunk low-fat cheese

Lunch

- Sliced steak (leftover London Broil) on mixed leaves
- 2 tablespoons Balsamic Vinaigrette (page 137) or 2 tablespoons low-sugar dressing
- Sugar-free jelly

Mid-afternoon snack

- Hummus (page 162) with raw vegetables (you may use ready-made hummus)

Dinner

- Savoury Chicken Sauté (page 142)
- Surprise South Beach Mashed 'Potatoes' (page 158)
- Fresh steamed green beans
- Round lettuce and pecan salad
- Olive oil and vinegar to taste

Dessert

- Vanilla Ricotta Crème (page 165)

DAY NINE

Breakfast

- 150ml (6 fl oz) vegetable juice cocktail
- 2 Vegetable Quiche Cups To Go (page 125)
- Decaffeinated coffee or decaffeinated tea with skimmed milk and sugar substitute

Mid-morning snack

- 1–2 Turkey Rolls (page 163)
- 2 tablespoons Coriander Mayonnaise (optional) (page 163)

Lunch

- Greek Salad (page 128)
- Sugar-free jelly

Mid-afternoon snack

- Celery stuffed with 1 wedge Laughing Cow Light Cheese

Dinner

- Fish Kebabs with Spaghetti Squash (pages 153 and 209)
- Sliced cucumber with olive oil

Dessert

- Lemon Zest Ricotta Crème (page 164)

DAY TEN

Breakfast

- 175ml (6 fl oz) tomato juice
- Egg white omelette with chopped lean bacon and mushrooms
- Decaffeinated coffee or decaffeinated tea with skimmed milk and sugar substitute

Mid-morning snack

- 1 wedge Laughing Cow Light Cheese

Lunch

- Salad Niçoise (page 136)

Mid-afternoon snack

- 75g (3 oz) low-fat cottage cheese

Dinner

- Cracked Pepper Steak (page 148)
- Grilled Tomato with Pesto (page 159)
- Steamed broccoli
- Mixed greens
- 2 tablespoons Balsamic Vinaigrette (page 137) or low-sugar prepared dressing

Dessert

- Almond Ricotta Crème (page 164)

DAY ELEVEN

Breakfast

- 175ml (6 fl oz) tomato juice
- Cheesy Frittata (page 120)
- Decaffeinated coffee or decaffeinated tea with skimmed milk and sugar substitute

Mid-morning snack

- 1–2 Turkey Roll-ups (page 163)
- 2 tablespoons Coriander Mayonnaise (optional) (page 163)

Lunch

- Gazpacho (page 138)
- Grilled sirloin hamburger steak (no bun)
- Tossed salad (mixed leaves, cucumber, green peppers, cherry tomatoes)
- Olive oil and vinegar to taste or 2 tablespoons low-sugar prepared dressing

Mid-afternoon snack

- Piece of fresh mozzarella cheese

Dinner

- Gingered Chicken Breast (page 141)
- Steamed mange-tout
- Oriental Cabbage Salad (page 161)

Dessert

- Almond Ricotta Crème (page 164)

DAY TWELVE

Breakfast

- 150ml (6 fl oz) vegetable juice cocktail
- Broccoli and Ham Frittata (page 122)
- Decaffeinated coffee or decaffeinated tea with skimmed milk and sugar substitute

Mid-morning snack

- 1 wedge Laughing Cow Light Cheese

Lunch

- Chicken-Pistachio Salad (page 131)

Mid-afternoon snack

- Piece of fresh mozzarella cheese

Dinner

- Poached Salmon with Cucumber-Dill Sauce (page 149)
- Edamame Salad (page 161)
- Grilled Tomatoes with Pesto (page 159)
- Steamed asparagus

Dessert

- Lemon Zest Ricotta Crème (page 164)

DAY THIRTEEN

Breakfast

- Baked eggs with lean, low-fat bacon strips
- Decaffeinated coffee or decaffeinated tea with skimmed milk and sugar substitute

Mid-morning snack

- Celery stuffed with 1 wedge Laughing Cow Light Cheese

Lunch

- Poached Salmon Spinach Salad (poached salmon left over from Day 12) (page 186)
- Olive oil and vinegar to taste or 2 tablespoons low-sugar prepared dressing

Mid-afternoon snack

- Hummus (page 162) with raw vegetables (you may use ready-made hummus)

Dinner

- Barbecued Steak with Tomato Relish (page 147)

Dessert

- Mocha Ricotta Crème (page 165)

DAY FOURTEEN

Breakfast

- Artichokes Benedict (page 126)
- Mock Hollandaise Sauce (page 127)
- Decaffeinated coffee or decaffeinated tea with skimmed milk and sugar substitute

Mid-morning snack

- 1–2 Turkey Roll-ups (page 163)
- 2 tablespoons Coriander Mayonnaise (optional) (page 163)

Lunch

- Red pepper stuffed with cottage cheese and chopped vegetables

Mid-afternoon snack

- Hummus (page 162) with raw vegetables (you may use ready-made hummus)

Dinner

- Grilled chicken breast with plain grilled vegetables and fennel or endive

Dessert

- Sugar-free jelly with a tablespoon of low-fat topping or whipping cream with sugar substitute to taste

Foods to Enjoy

BEEF
Sirloin (including minced)
Tenderloin
Top round
Other lean cuts

POULTRY (SKINLESS)
Turkey and chicken breast
Poussin
Turkey bacon (2 slices per day)

SEAFOOD
All types of fish and shellfish

PORK
Boiled ham
Lean bacon
Tenderloin

VEAL
Leg cutlet
Top round
Veal chop

LUNCHMEAT
Nonfat or lower fat only

CHEESE (FAT-FREE OR LOWER FAT)
American
Cheddar
Feta
Mozzarella
Parmesan
Ricotta
Provolone

String
Dairy-free cream cheese substitute
1–2% or fat-free cottage cheese

NUTS
30 pistachios
20 small peanuts
15 pecan halves
1 teaspoon peanut butter

EGGS
The use of whole eggs is not limited unless otherwise directed by your doctor.
Use of egg whites as desired.

TOFU
Use soft, low-fat, or lite varieties

VEGETABLES
Alfalfa sprouts
Artichokes
Asparagus
Aubergines
Beans (black, butter, chickpeas, green, Italian, kidney, lentils, lima, pigeon, soy, split peas and wax)
Broccoli
Cabbage
Cauliflower
Celery
Collard greens
Courgettes
Cucumbers
Lettuce (all varieties)
Mushrooms (all varieties)

Snow peas
Spinach
Turnips
Water chestnuts

FATS
Canola oil
Olive oil

SPICES AND SEASONINGS
All spices that contain no added sugar
Broth
Extracts (almond, vanilla, etc.)

Horseradish sauce
Low-fat butter substitute
Pepper – black, cayenne, red, white

SWEET TREATS
Limit to 75 calories per day
Baking cocoa powder
No-added-sugar chocolate powder
Sugar-free ice-lollies
Sugar-free gelatin
Sugar-free hard sweets
Sugarless chewing gum
Sugar substitute

Foods to Avoid

BEEF
Brisket
Liver
Other fatty cuts
Rib steaks

POULTRY
Chicken wings and legs
Duck
Goose
Processed poultry products

PORK
Honey-baked ham

VEAL
Veal breast

CHEESE
Brie
Edam
Nonreduced fat

VEGETABLES
Beets
Carrots
Corn
Potatoes
Tomato (limit to 1 whole or 10 cherry per meal)
Sweet potatoes
Yams

FRUIT
Avoid all fruits and fruit juices in Phase 1, including:
Apples
Apricots
Berries
Cantaloupe
Grapefruit
Peaches
Pears

STARCHES AND CARBS
Avoid all starchy food in Phase 1, including:
Bread, all types
Cereal
Oatmeal
Rice, all types
Pasta, all types
Pastry and baked goods, all types

DAIRY
Avoid all dairy in Phase 1, including:
Frozen yogurt
Ice-cream
Milk
Soya milk
Yogurt

MISCELLANEOUS
Alcohol of any kind, including beer and wine

chapter fourteen

phase 1 recipes

Because this is the strictest phase, the palette of ingredients is relatively small. You'll be eating eggs for breakfast and lots of vegetables, low-fat cheeses, meat and fish the rest of the time. There's no bread, potatoes, fruit or rice during the first 2 weeks, true. But any plan that permits dishes such as Marinated Rump Steak, Crab Cobb Salad, Hummus and Lemon Zest Ricotta Crème can hardly be termed tough. And any programme that requires you to eat 6 times a day – 3 meals plus snacks in mid-morning and mid-afternoon, plus a nighttime dessert – is clearly meant to keep discomfort to a minimum.

BREAKFASTS

CHEESY FRITTATA

Serves 2

Lite cooking spray
2 teaspoons healthy butter-substitute spread
50g (2 oz) sliced onion
50g (2 oz) sliced red pepper
50g (2 oz) sliced courgette
2 small plum tomatoes, diced
1 tablespoon chopped fresh basil
Pinch freshly ground black pepper
2 eggs
100g (4 oz) virtually fat-free cottage cheese
50ml (2 fl oz) fat-free evaporated milk
20g (1¾ oz) grated reduced-fat Cheddar cheese

Coat an ovenproof 30cm (10-inch) frying pan with cooking spray and place over medium-low heat until hot. In the frying pan, melt the spread. Add the onion, red pepper, and courgette and sauté over medium-low heat until the vegetables are lightly browned, 2–3 minutes. Add the tomatoes, basil, and black pepper to the frying pan and stir to combine. Cook until the flavours are blended, 2–3 minutes, and remove from the heat.

Preheat the grill. In a blender, combine the eggs, cottage cheese, and milk and process until smooth. Pour the egg mixture over the vegetables. Cover and cook on medium-low heat until the bottom is set and the top is still slightly wet. Transfer the pan to the grill and grill until the top is set, 2–3 minutes. Sprinkle with the cheese and grill until the cheese melts.

Nutrition at a Glance

Per serving: 231 calories, 21g protein, 16g carbohydrates, 10g fat, 3g saturated fat, 480g sodium, 15mg cholesterol, 2g fibre

LIGHT SPINACH FRITTATA WITH TOMATO SALSA

Serves 2

Frittata

- 1 tablespoon extra-virgin olive oil
- 1 small onion, sliced
- 2 cloves garlic, finely chopped
- 300g (10 oz) frozen spinach, thawed and well-drained
- 2 large eggs
- 3 egg whites
- 75ml (2½ fl oz) light evaporated milk
- 100g (4 oz) grated reduced-fat mozzarella cheese

Salsa

- 4 plum tomatoes, seeded and chopped
- 2 spring onions, finely chopped
- 1 clove garlic, finely chopped
- 2 tablespoons finely chopped fresh coriander
- 1 tablespoon fresh lime juice
- ¼ teaspoon salt
- ⅛ teaspoon freshly ground black pepper

To make the frittata: Preheat the oven to 180°C/350°F/Gas 4. Heat the oil in a 25cm (10-inch) non-stick ovenproof frying pan over medium heat. Add the onion and garlic and cook, stirring, for 3 minutes or until tender. Stir in the spinach. Reduce the heat to low. In a large bowl, beat the eggs and egg whites with the milk until light yellow and frothy. Pour the egg mixture over the spinach in the frying pan. Cook for 5–7 minutes, until the egg mixture is cooked on the bottom and almost set on top. Sprinkle with the cheese. Bake in the oven until the eggs are set and the cheese has melted, 5–10 minutes.

To make the salsa: In a large bowl, stir together the tomatoes, spring onions, garlic, coriander, lime juice, salt, and pepper. Serve fresh at room temperature over the frittata.

You can also serve the frittata with ready-made salsa.

Nutrition at a Glance

Per serving: 369 calories, 27g protein, 28g carbohydrates, 17g fat, 6g saturated fat, 740mg sodium, 230mg cholesterol, 8g fibre

SMOKED SALMON FRITTATA

Serves 2

8 spears fresh asparagus
Lite cooking spray
1 tablespoon extra-virgin olive oil
½ Spanish onion
50g (2 oz) dry-packed sun-dried tomatoes
50g (2 oz) smoked salmon
2 eggs
50ml (2 fl oz) water
3 tablespoons skimmed powdered milk
¼ teaspoon chopped fresh marjoram
Pinch freshly ground black pepper

Bring 2cm (1 inch) water to a boil in a large frying pan. Add the asparagus and cook, uncovered, just until tender. Coat an ovenproof 20cm (8-inch) frying pan with non-stick cooking spray and place over medium-low heat until hot. Add the olive oil and sauté the onion until soft. Add the asparagus and sun-dried tomatoes. Add the smoked salmon and remove from the heat. Preheat the grill. Combine the eggs, water, powdered milk, marjoram, and pepper. Pour over the salmon mixture. Cover and cook over medium-low heat for 7 minutes or until the bottom is set and the top is slightly wet. Place the frying pan under the grill 10–14cm (4–6 inches) from the heat source until the top of the frittata is puffed and set, 2–3 minutes. Top with fat-free sour cream and chives if desired. Slice into wedges and serve immediately.

For variety you can substitute broccoli and ham for the asparagus and salmon if you wish.

Nutrition at a Glance

Per serving: 241 calories, 19g protein, 18g carbohydrates, 11g fat, 2g saturated fat, 730mg sodium, 5mg cholesterol, 4g fibre

EASY ASPARAGUS AND MUSHROOM OMELETTE

Serves 1

3 stalks fresh asparagus
2 eggs
2 tablespoons water
Lite cooking spray
50g (2 oz) sliced white mushrooms
50g (2 oz) grated reduced-fat mozzarella cheese

Bring 2cm (1 inch) water to a boil in a large frying pan. Add the asparagus and cook, uncovered, just until tender. Meanwhile, in a medium bowl, whisk together the eggs and water. The whites and the yolk should be blended completely together.

Coat a 25cm (10-inch) non-stick frying pan with cooking spray. Heat the frying pan over medium-high heat until just hot enough to sizzle when a drop of water is added. Pour in the egg mixture. It should set immediately. With a spatula, lift edges as mixture begins to set to allow uncooked portion to flow underneath. When top is set, fill one half of the omelette with asparagus, mushrooms, and cheese. With the spatula, fold the omelette in half over the filling. Slide onto a serving plate. Serve immediately.

Nutrition at a Glance

Per serving: 238 calories, 21g protein, 5g carbohydrates, 15g fat, 6g saturated fat, 260mg sodium, 440mg cholesterol, 1g fibre

WESTERN EGG WHITE OMELETTE

Serves 1

Lite cooking spray
1 tablespoon chopped green pepper
1 tablespoon chopped spring onion
1 tablespoon chopped red pepper
2 eggs
3 tablespoons grated reduced-fat cheese

Lightly coat a medium frying pan with cooking spray. Sauté the green pepper, spring onion, and red pepper until they are slightly tender. Pour the eggs over the vegetables. When partially set, spread the cheese over half of the egg and fold the omelette. Continue cooking until cooked through.

Nutrition at a Glance

Per serving: 169 calories, 20g protein, 4g carbohydrates, 8g fat, 3g saturated fat, 320mg sodium, 15mg cholesterol, 1g fibre

VEGETABLE QUICHE CUPS TO GO

Serves 6

300g (10 oz) frozen chopped spinach
3 eggs
100g (4 oz) grated reduced-fat cheese
50g (2 oz) finely chopped green peppers
50g (2 oz) finely chopped onions
3 drops Tabasco sauce (optional)

Microwave the spinach for 2½ minutes on high. Drain excess liquid.

Line 12 muffin tins with baking cases.

Combine the eggs, cheese, peppers, onions, spinach, and Tabasco sauce if using, in a bowl. Mix well. Divide evenly among the muffin cases. Bake at 180°C/350°F/Gas 4 for 20 minutes until a knife inserted in the centre comes out clean.

Quiche cups can be frozen and reheated in the microwave. Any combination of appropriate vegetables and reduced-fat cheeses may be used.

Nutrition at a Glance

Per serving: 77 calories, 9g protein, 3g carbohydrates, 3g fat, 2g saturated fat, 160mg sodium, 10mg cholesterol, 2g fibre

ARTICHOKES BENEDICT

Serves 2

2 medium globe artichokes
2 slices lean bacon
2 eggs
4 tablespoons Mock Hollandaise Sauce (see opposite)

Wash the artichokes. Cut off the stems at the base and remove the small bottom leaves. Stand the artichokes upright in a deep saucepan with 5–7cm (2–3 inches) salted water. Cover and boil gently, 35–45 minutes. Turn the artichokes upside down to drain. Spread the leaves open like flower petals. With a spoon, carefully remove the centre petals and the fuzzy centre from the artichoke bottoms and discard. Keep the artichokes warm. Brown the bacon in a frying pan and poach the eggs in boiling salted water. Place a bacon slice into each artichoke top with a poached egg and Mock Hollandaise Sauce. Serve immediately.

Nutrition at a Glance

Per serving: 227 calories, 18g protein, 16g carbohydrates, 12g fat, 3g saturated fat, 540mg sodium, 225mg cholesterol, 8g fibre

MOCK HOLLANDAISE SAUCE

Serves 2

1 egg
1 tablespoon healthy butter-substitute spread
1 teaspoon fresh lemon juice
½ teaspoon Dijon mustard
Pinch paprika

In a 10 fl oz (½ pint) microwaveable liquid measure, combine the egg and the spread. Microwave on low (20%) for 1 minute, stirring once halfway through cooking, until the spread is softened.

Stir the lemon juice and mustard into the egg mixture and microwave on low for 3 minutes, stirring every 30 seconds, until thickened. Stir in the paprika. (If the mixture curdles, transfer to a blender and process on low speed for 30 seconds, until smooth.)

Nutrition at a Glance

Per serving: 54 calories, 4g protein, 2g carbohydrates, 4g fat, 0g saturated fat, 150mg sodium, 5mg cholesterol, 0g fibre

LUNCHES

GREEK SALAD

Serves 1

8 lettuce leaves, torn into bite-size pieces
1 cucumber, peeled, seeded, and sliced
1 tomato, chopped
50g (2 oz) sliced red onion
50g (2 oz) crumbled reduced-fat feta cheese
2 tablespoons extra-virgin olive oil
2 tablespoons fresh lemon juice
1 teaspoon dried oregano leaves
½ teaspoon salt

Combine the lettuce, cucumber, tomato, onion, and cheese in a large bowl.
   Whisk together the oil, lemon juice, oregano, and salt in a small bowl.
Pour over the lettuce mixture and toss until coated.
   This makes a nice accompaniment as a side salad for grilled chicken or fish.

Nutrition at a Glance

Per serving: 501 calories, 22g protein, 25g carbohydrates, 38g fat, 10g saturated fat, 2300mg sodium (1134mg if salt omitted), 30mg cholesterol, 6g fibre

CHERRY SNAPPER CEVICHE*

(Phase I Lunch or Dinner)

Serves 4

4 cherry snapper or trout fillets, coarsely chopped
3 fresh limes, juice of
½ teaspoon red chilli garlic paste (sambal oelek)
2 ripe plum tomatoes, coarsely chopped
½ yellow Spanish onion, coarsely chopped
2½ tablespoons fresh coriander, finely chopped
Sea salt
Black pepper

Soak the chopped fish in ¾ of the lime juice for 3 hours. Drain off the liquid and discard. Mix the fish with the red chilli garlic paste, tomatoes, onion, coriander, and the remaining lime juice. Season with salt and pepper to taste.

Nutrition at a Glance

Per serving: 225 calories, 36g protein, 15g carbohydrates, 2g fat, 1g saturated fat, 115mg sodium, 63mg cholesterol, 3g fibre

SOUTH BEACH CHOPPED SALAD WITH TUNA

Serves 1

Salad

1 tin tuna chunks in brine (185g/6½ oz), drained and flaked
75g (3 oz) chopped cucumber
75g (3 oz) chopped tomato
75g (3 oz) chopped avocado
75g (3 oz) chopped celery
75g (3 oz) chopped radishes
1 handful chopped romaine lettuce

Dressing

4 teaspoons extra-virgin olive oil
2 tablespoons fresh lime juice
2 cloves garlic, finely chopped
½ teaspoon crushed black pepper

To make the salad: Layer the tuna, cucumber, tomato, avocado, celery, radishes, and lettuce in a decorative glass bowl.

To make the dressing: Mix the olive oil, lime juice, garlic, and pepper. Drizzle over the salad.

Nutrition at a Glance

Per serving: 506 calories, 48g protein, 18g carbohydrates, 28g fat, 4g saturated fat, 640mg sodium, 50mg cholesterol, 6g fibre

CHICKEN-PISTACHIO SALAD

Serves 4

Salad

50g (2 oz) shelled pistachio nuts, finely ground
½ + ¼ teaspoon salt
½ teaspoon + 1 pinch freshly ground black pepper
4 boneless, skinless chicken breast halves
2 tablespoons extra-virgin olive oil
50g (2 oz) chopped sweet white onion
1 head romaine lettuce

Dressing

1 teaspoon grated sweet white onion
1 large ripe avocado, pitted and peeled
3 tablespoons extra-virgin olive oil
3 tablespoons fresh lime juice
1 tablespoon water

To make the salad: Preheat the oven to 190°C/375°F/Gas 5. Mix the nuts with ½ teaspoon salt and ½ teaspoon pepper in a pie dish. Press the chicken into the nuts. Heat 1 tablespoon of oil in a frying pan and cook the coated breasts, 2 minutes per side. Place the breasts in a baking dish, place in the oven, and bake for 15 minutes or until a thermometer inserted in the thickest portion registers 71°C (160°F) and the juices run clear.

Heat the remaining tablespoon of oil in a non-stick frying pan over high heat. Add the chopped onion, ¼ teaspoon salt, and a pinch of pepper. Cook until the onion is browned. Line 4 serving plates with lettuce.

To make the dressing: Purée the onion, avocado, oil, lime juice, and water in a blender.

Slice the chicken breasts and arrange 1 breast on top of the lettuce on each plate. Serve with the dressing.

Nutrition at a Glance

Per serving: 481 calories, 33g protein, 13g carbohydrates, 34g fat, 5g saturated fat, 520mg sodium, 70mg cholesterol, 5g fibre

DILLED PRAWN SALAD WITH HERB-DILL DRESSING

Serves 4

Prawns

225ml (8 fl oz) dry white wine

1 teaspoon mustard seeds

¼ teaspoon crushed red pepper

2 bay leaves

1 lemon, sliced

700g (1½ lb) large uncooked prawns (peeled and deveined)

Herb-Dill Dressing

3 tablespoons extra-virgin olive oil	1 teaspoon Dijon mustard
3 tablespoons red wine vinegar	½ medium onion, sliced
2 tablespoons water	1 large head romaine lettuce
2 tablespoons chopped fresh basil	4 ripe tomatoes, cut into wedges
2 tablespoons chopped fresh dill	6 fresh mushrooms, sliced
1 teaspoon finely chopped garlic	Fresh dill sprigs (optional)

To prepare the prawns: Combine the wine, mustard seeds, crushed pepper, bay leaves, and lemon in a large saucepan. Add water to fill pan two-thirds full. Bring to a boil over high heat, add prawns, and cook for 3–4 minutes or until prawns have turned pink and are no longer translucent in the centre. Drain and cool. Discard the bay leaves.

To make the herb-dill dressing: In a screw-top jar, mix the olive oil, red wine vinegar, water, basil, dill, garlic, mustard, and onion. Shake well.

Place the prawns in a large bowl and add the dressing. Toss well, cover, and refrigerate until well chilled. Serve the prawn mixture on romaine lettuce leaves and surround with tomato wedges and mushroom slices. Garnish with dill sprigs, if using.

Nutrition at a Glance

Per serving: 382 calories, 38g protein, 16g carbohydrates, 14g fat, 2g saturated fat, 310mg sodium, 260mg cholesterol, 4g fibre

CRAB COBB SALAD

Serves 2

6 handfuls romaine lettuce, torn into bite-size pieces
I tin crabmeat (185g/6½ oz), drained
225g (8 oz) chopped ripe tomatoes or halved cherry tomatoes
50g (2 oz) crumbled blue cheese
2 tablespoons cholesterol-free bacon bits e.g. Bacos
50ml (2 fl oz) prepared low-sugar dressing or olive oil vinaigrette

Arrange the lettuce on a large serving dish. Arrange the crabmeat, tomatoes, blue cheese, and bacon bits in rows over the lettuce. Just before serving, drizzle some dressing evenly over the salad and toss well. Transfer to 2 chilled serving plates.

Nutrition at a Glance

Per serving: 267 calories, 27g protein, 12g carbohydrates, 13g fat, 4g saturated fat, 1012mg sodium, 95mg cholesterol, 4g fibre

SPICY TUNA*

(Phase I Dinner)

Serves 4

50g (2 oz) white pepper
50g (2 oz) black pepper
50g (2 oz) fennel seeds
50g (2 oz) coriander seeds
50g (2 oz) ground cumin
2 tuna fillets (225g/8 oz each)
4 egg yolks
2½ tablespoons fresh coriander
2½ tablespoons fresh chives
2½ tablespoons parsley
4 deseeded green chillis
225ml (8 fl oz) rice vinegar
350ml (12 fl oz) olive oil
3 roasted red peppers
1 cucumber, finely sliced

In a preheated oven at 170°C/325°F/Gas 3, roast the white pepper, black pepper, fennel, and coriander for 15 minutes. Mix with the cumin and grind in a blender until finely ground.

Coat the tuna well with the roasted spices and pan sear until medium-rare. Set aside.

Make a chilli vinaigrette in a blender by mixing 2 of the egg yolks with the coriander, chives, parsley, and chillis and 100ml (4 fl oz) of rice vinegar. Add 150ml (6 fl oz) of oil slowly to emulsify.

Make a roasted pepper vinaigrette in a blender by mixing the remaining 2 egg yolks with the remaining 100ml (4 fl oz) of rice vinegar and the roasted red peppers, then emulsifying with the remaining oil.

Place the chilli vinaigrette and the roasted pepper vinaigrette on each half of a large dish. Slice the tuna and place on top of the vinaigrette. Garnish with the cucumber.

Nutrition at a Glance

Per serving: 626 calories, 37g protein, 57g carbohydrates, 26g fat, 4g unsaturated fat, 137mg sodium, 266mg cholesterol, 21g fibre

MIXED GREENS

150g (5 oz) torn curly endive
150g (5 oz) loosely packed watercress leaves
150g (5 oz) torn fresh spinach
150g (5 oz) torn red leaf cabbage
75g (3 oz) sliced water chestnuts
1 red pepper, sliced into strips
350g (12 oz) crabmeat, fresh or canned
Joe's Mustard Sauce (page 160)

Combine the vegetables in a large bowl. Toss well. Add the crabmeat. Divide onto 4 serving plates, drizzle Joe's Mustard Sauce on top.

Nutrition at a Glance

Per serving: 123 calories, 20g protein, 9g carbohydrates, 1g fat, 0g saturated fat, 338mg sodium, 76mg cholesterol, 4g fibre

SALAD NIÇOISE

Serves 4

225g (½ lb) tiny green beans
225g (½ lb) tiny ripe tomatoes, cut into wedges
1 green pepper, seeded and cut into strips
1 cucumber, cut into thick strips
55g (2 oz) tinned anchovies, drained
110g (4 oz) pitted black olives
1 tin tuna chunks in brine (185g/6½ oz), drained and flaked
110g (4 oz) sliced water chestnuts
4 hard-boiled eggs, shelled and quartered
5 tablespoons extra-virgin olive oil
1 tablespoon white wine vinegar
1 clove garlic, finely chopped
Pinch salt
Pinch freshly ground black pepper
2 tablespoons finely chopped fresh flat-leaf parsley

Blanch the beans briefly until just tender and refresh in cold running water.
Pat dry. Mix the tomatoes, pepper, and cucumber in a large salad bowl (or
arrange in separate piles around the inside of the bowl). Arrange the
anchovies, olives, tuna, water chestnuts, and eggs over the top. Make a
dressing by vigorously mixing the oil, vinegar, and garlic with the salt and
pepper. Pour the dressing over the salad and sprinkle with the parsley.

Nutrition at a Glance

Per serving: 405 calories, 26g protein, 14g carbohydrates, 27g fat, 5g
saturated fat, 1010mg sodium, 240mg cholesterol, 4g fibre

BALSAMIC VINAIGRETTE

Makes 150ml (5 fl oz)

75ml (3 fl oz) extra-virgin olive oil
75ml (3 fl oz) balsamic vinegar
2 teaspoons chopped fresh thyme
¼ teaspoon salt
⅛ teaspoon white pepper
1 tablespoon chopped fresh basil

Combine the olive oil, vinegar, thyme, salt, pepper, and basil in a screw-top jar. Cover and shake.

Nutrition at a Glance

Per serving: 90 calories, 0g protein, 2g carbohydrates, 9g fat, 1g saturated fat, 75mg sodium, 0mg cholesterol, 0g fibre

GAZPACHO

Serves 5

600ml (1 pint) tomato or vegetable juice
225g (8 oz) peeled, seeded, finely chopped fresh tomatoes
110g (4 oz) finely chopped celery
110g (4 oz) finely chopped cucumber
110g (4 oz) finely chopped green pepper
110g (4 oz) finely chopped spring onions
3 tablespoons white wine vinegar
2 tablespoons extra-virgin olive oil
1 large clove garlic, finely chopped
2 teaspoons finely chopped fresh flat-leaf parsley
½ teaspoon salt
½ teaspoon Worcestershire sauce
½ teaspoon freshly ground black pepper

Combine the juice, tomatoes, celery, cucumber, pepper, onions, vinegar, oil, garlic, parsley, salt, Worcestershire sauce, and black pepper in a large glass or stainless-steel bowl. Cover and refrigerate overnight. Serve cold.

Nutrition at a Glance

Per serving: 117 calories, 2g protein, 13g carbohydrates, 6g fat, 1g saturated fat, 690mg sodium, 0mg cholesterol, 4g fibre

DINNERS

CHICKEN EN PAPILLOTE

Serves 4

4 boneless, skinless chicken breast halves (about 500g/1 lb)
Pinch salt
Pinch freshly ground black pepper
2 spring onions, chopped
1 medium carrot, sliced diagonally
1 small courgette, cut lengthwise in half, then crosswise into 1cm
  (½-inch) thick pieces
1 teaspoon dried tarragon
½ teaspoon grated orange zest

Heat oven to 200°C/400°F/Gas 6 (220°C/425°F/Gas 7 if foil is used). Cut four 60cm (2-foot) lengths of baking parchment or foil and fold each in half to make a 30cm (1-foot) square. Sprinkle the chicken breasts with salt and pepper. Place a breast slightly below the middle of each square of paper.

In a small bowl, combine the spring onions, carrot, courgette, tarragon, and orange zest. Spoon a quarter of the vegetable mixture over each chicken breast.

Fold the parchment or foil over the chicken, crimp edges together tightly, and bake for 20 minutes on a baking sheet. To serve, cut an X in the top of each packet with scissors and tear open.

Nutrition at a Glance

Per serving: 144 calories, 27g protein, 4g carbohydrates, 2g fat, 0g saturated fat, 86mg sodium, 65mg cholesterol, 1g fibre

BALSAMIC CHICKEN

Serves 6

6 boneless, skinless chicken breast halves
1½ teaspoons fresh rosemary leaves, finely chopped, or ½ teaspoon
    dried rosemary
2 cloves garlic, finely chopped
½ teaspoon freshly ground black pepper
½ teaspoon salt
2 tablespoons extra-virgin olive oil
Lite cooking spray
4–6 tablespoons white wine (optional)
75ml (3 fl oz) balsamic vinegar

Rinse the chicken and pat dry. Combine the rosemary, garlic, pepper, and salt in a small bowl; mix well. Place the chicken in a large bowl; drizzle with oil, and rub with the spice mixture. Cover and refrigerate overnight.

Preheat the oven to 230°C/450°F/Gas 8. Spray a heavy roasting pan or cast-iron frying pan with cooking spray. Place the chicken in the pan and bake for 10 minutes. Turn the chicken over, stirring in 3–4 tablespoons water or white wine (if using) if drippings begin to stick to the pan.

Bake for about 10 minutes or until a thermometer inserted in the thickest portion registers 71°C (160°F) and the juices run clear. If the pan is dry, stir in another 1–2 tablespoons of water or white wine to loosen drippings.

Drizzle the vinegar over the chicken in the pan. Transfer the chicken to plates. Stir the liquid in the pan; drizzle over the chicken.

Nutrition at a Glance

Per serving: 183 calories, 26g protein, 4g carbohydrates, 6g fat, 1g saturated fat, 270mg sodium, 65mg cholesterol, 0g fibre

GINGERED CHICKEN BREASTS

Serves 4

1 tablespoon fresh lemon juice
1½ teaspoons grated fresh ginger
½ teaspoon freshly ground black pepper
2 cloves garlic
4 boneless, skinless chicken breast halves
Lite cooking spray

Combine the lemon juice, ginger, pepper, and garlic in a small bowl. Place the chicken breasts in a deep bowl, pour on the ginger mixture, turn once to coat both sides, cover, and refrigerate for 30 minutes to 2 hours.

Spray a large non-stick frying pan with cooking spray. Heat the frying pan on medium-high heat until hot. Add the chicken and cook, turning once, until tender, about 8 minutes.

Nutrition at a Glance

Per serving: 129 calories, 26g protein, 1g carbohydrates, 1g fat, 0g saturated fat, 75mg sodium, 65mg cholesterol, 0g fibre

SAVOURY CHICKEN SAUTÉ

Serves 4

2 tablespoons extra-virgin olive oil
4 boneless, skinless chicken breast halves
1 large onion, sliced
2 cloves garlic, finely chopped
1 tablespoon fresh rosemary leaves, chopped
100ml (4 fl oz) fat-free chicken stock
Pinch salt
Pinch freshly ground black pepper

Heat the oil in a large frying pan over medium heat. Sauté the chicken breasts in the oil for 4 minutes, then turn them over and add the onion. Cover and cook 3 minutes longer, stirring occasionally. Add the garlic, rosemary, and stock. Cover and cook until the onion starts to brown and about 5 minutes longer, stirring occasionally. Season with salt and pepper.

Nutrition at a Glance

Per serving: 217 calories, 28g protein, 6g carbohydrates, 8g fat, 1g saturated fat, 95mg sodium, 65mg cholesterol, 1g fibre

FLORENTINE-STYLE T-BONE*

(Phase I Dinner)

Serves 4

1.6kg (3½ lb) prime T-bone steak
2 tablespoons finely chopped fresh garlic
25g (1 oz) chopped parsley
25g (1 oz) chopped basil
Salt
Freshly ground black pepper
225ml (8 fl oz) extra-virgin olive oil

Season the steak with garlic, parsley, and basil and salt and pepper to taste. Drizzle it with the olive oil and marinate for 24 hours. When ready to cook, heat the grill or barbecue and cook on medium heat, turning every 10 minutes for a total of 1 hour. While cooking, preheat the oven to 200°C/400°F/Gas 6. Once the meat is ready, let it stand for 20 minutes. Roast in the oven for 10 to 30 minutes, depending on how you like your meat. One hour under the grill or on the barbecue and 10 minutes in the oven will yield a medium-rare meat. A meat thermometer should register 63°C (145°F) for medium-rare.

Slice the steak and drizzle with some of the olive oil marinade (now at room temperature).

Nutrition at a Glance

Per serving: 885 calories, 59g protein, 5g carbohydrates, 68g fat, 13g saturated fat, 170mg sodium, 105mg cholesterol, 1g fibre

MARINATED RUMP STEAK

Serves 6

1 small red onion
75ml (3 fl oz) balsamic vinegar
50g (2 oz) capers, drained
2 tablespoons chopped fresh oregano
3 cloves garlic, finely chopped
700g (1½ lb) rump steak
¼ teaspoon salt
¼ teaspoon coarsely ground black pepper

Sliver one-quarter of the onion and set aside. Chop the rest of the onion. In a bowl, mix the chopped onion, vinegar, capers, oregano, and garlic. Sprinkle both sides of the steak with salt and pepper; prick well with a fork. Mix half of the onion mixture with the slivered onions. In a large zip-top food-storage bag, combine the steak with the remaining mixture. Marinate for 1 hour or overnight. Prepare the barbecue for direct heat or position the grill tray so that the meat on the tray in the pan is 10cm (4 inches) from the heat source; heat the grill. Remove the meat from the marinade, discarding the marinade. Place on the barbecue or on the grill tray. Grill or barbecue for 4–5 minutes per side for medium-rare. Let stand for 5 minutes before slicing. Place the meat on a dish and pour the reserved onion over the steak.

Nutrition at a Glance

Per serving: 176 calories, 19g protein, 3g carbohydrates, 9g fat, 4g saturated fat, 230mg sodium, 50mg cholesterol, 1g fibre

GRILLED RUMP STEAK

Serves 4

1 rump steak (500g/1 ½ lb)
100ml (4 fl oz) tomato juice
50ml (2 fl oz) Worcestershire sauce
1 small onion, finely chopped
1 tablespoon fresh lemon juice
1 clove garlic, finely chopped
½ teaspoon freshly ground black pepper
⅛ teaspoon salt

Place the steak in a 32 × 22cm (13 × 9 inch) glass baking dish. Combine the tomato juice, Worcestershire sauce, onion, lemon juice, garlic, pepper, and salt and pour over the steak. Cover and refrigerate for 2 hours, turning once.

Place the steak on the grill tray and brush with marinade. Grill 7cm (3 inches) from heat for 5 minutes. Turn, brush with marinade, and grill for 3 minutes or until a thermometer inserted in the centre registers 63°C (145°F) for medium-rare.

To serve, cut diagonally across grain into thin slices.

Nutrition at a Glance

Per serving: 265 calories, 29g protein, 6g carbohydrates, 13g fat, 6g saturated fat, 440mg sodium, 70mg cholesterol, 0g fibre

MARINATED LONDON BROIL

Serves 8

2 tablespoons extra-virgin olive oil
100ml (4 fl oz) dry red wine
3 cloves garlic, finely chopped
3 tablespoons finely chopped fresh parsley
1 tablespoon chopped fresh oregano
1 bay leaf
½ teaspoon freshly ground black pepper
700g (1½ lb) sirloin or rump steak

In a small mixing bowl, whisk together the oil, wine, garlic, parsley, oregano, bay leaf, and pepper. Place the steak in a deep bowl, pour on the marinade, turn once to coat both sides, cover, and refrigerate for at least 4 hours, preferably overnight. Preheat the grill or prepare a barbecue. Discard the marinade and bay leaf. Grill the meat for about 5 minutes on each side or until a thermometer inserted in the centre registers 63°C (145°F) for medium-rare. Cut the meat into thin, diagonal slices across the grain. Serve warm or cold.

Nutrition at a Glance

Per serving: 171 calories, 17g protein, 1g carbohydrates, 10g fat, 3g saturated fat, 50mg sodium, 40mg cholesterol, 0g fibre

BARBECUED STEAK WITH TOMATO RELISH

Serves 2

2 sirloin steaks (150g/6 oz each)
2 medium plum tomatoes, halved lengthwise
2 tablespoons extra-virgin olive oil
1 medium onion, chopped
1 clove garlic, finely chopped or pressed
20g (1 oz) chopped fresh basil or 2 tablespoons dry basil
Pinch salt
Pinch freshly ground black pepper
Basil sprigs (optional)

Place the steak on a lightly greased barbecue 10–15cm (4–6 inches) above a solid bed of medium-hot coals. Cook, turning as needed, until evenly browned on the outside and a thermometer inserted in the centre registers 63°C (145°F) for medium-rare; cut to test (about 15 minutes).

Meanwhile, place the tomatoes, cut side up, on the barbecue grill and brush lightly with 1 tablespoon of the oil. When the tomatoes are browned on the bottom (about 3 minutes), turn over and continue to cook until soft when pressed (about 3 more minutes).

While the tomatoes are cooking, combine the remaining 1 tablespoon oil, onion, and garlic in a medium frying pan with a heatproof handle. Set the pan over the coals (or set on the hob over medium-high heat). Cook, stirring often, until the onion is limp and golden (about 10 minutes); stir in the basil.

When the tomatoes are soft, stir them into the onion mixture, then set the pan aside on a cooler area of the barbecue (or cover and keep warm in the oven).

When the steak is done, place it on a board with a well (or on a dish); spoon tomato relish alongside steak. Season with salt and pepper and garnish with basil sprigs, if using. To serve, cut meat into thin slices. Spoon accumulated meat juices into tomato relish, if desired.

Nutrition at a Glance

Per serving: 366 calories, 31g protein, 11g carbohydrates, 22g fat, 5g saturated fat, 70mg sodium, 85mg cholesterol, 3g fibre

CRACKED PEPPER STEAK

Serves 2

1 tablespoon cracked black pepper
½ teaspoon dried rosemary
2 beef fillet steaks, 2.5cm (1 inch) thick (100–150g/4–6 oz each)
1 tablespoon healthy butter-substitute spread
1 tablespoon extra-virgin olive oil
50ml (2 fl oz) brandy or dry red wine

Combine the pepper and the rosemary in a large bowl. Coat both sides of the steak with the mixture.

Heat the spread and oil in a frying pan until hot. Add the steaks and cook over medium to medium-high heat for 5–7 minutes or until a thermometer inserted in the centre registers 70°C (160°F) for medium.

Remove the steaks from the frying pan and cover to keep warm.

Add the brandy or wine to the frying pan and bring to a boil over high heat, scraping particles from the bottom of the pan. Boil for about 1 minute or until the liquid is reduced by half. Spoon the sauce over the steaks.

Nutrition at a Glance

Per serving: 322 calories, 24g protein, 3g carbohydrates, 21g fat, 6g saturated fat, 55mg sodium, 70mg cholesterol, 1g fibre

POACHED SALMON WITH CUCUMBER-DILL SAUCE

Serves 6

Salmon
450ml (16 fl oz) Chablis or other dry white wine
450ml (16 fl oz) water
½ teaspoon chicken-flavoured bouillon granules
6 peppercorns
4 sprigs fresh dill
2 bay leaves
1 stalk celery, chopped
1 small lemon, sliced
6 salmon fillets, 1cm (½ inch) thick (100g/4 oz each)

Cucumber-Dill Sauce
75ml (3 fl oz) peeled, seeded, finely chopped cucumber
75ml (3 fl oz) fat-free sour cream
75ml (3 fl oz) fat-free plain yogurt
2 teaspoons chopped fresh dill
1 teaspoon Dijon mustard
Fresh dill sprigs (optional)

To cook the salmon: Combine the wine, water, bouillon, peppercorns, dill, bay leaves, celery, and lemon in a frying pan. Bring to a boil; cover, reduce heat, and simmer for 10 minutes. Add the salmon to the mixture in the frying pan and cook for 10 minutes or until the fish flakes easily. Transfer the salmon to a dish, using a slotted spoon; cover, and chill thoroughly. Discard the liquid mixture remaining in the frying pan.

To make the cucumber-dill sauce: In a medium bowl, mix together the cucumber, sour cream, yogurt, dill, and mustard.

To serve, place fillets on individual serving plates; spoon sauce evenly over fillets. Garnish with fresh dill sprigs, if using.

Nutrition at a Glance

Per serving: 260 calories, 24g protein, 5g carbohydrates, 13g fat, 3g saturated fat, 150mg sodium, 70mg cholesterol, 0g fibre

GRILLED SALMON WITH ROSEMARY

Serves 4

450g (1 lb) salmon
2 teaspoons extra-virgin olive oil
2 teaspoons fresh lemon juice
¼ teaspoon salt
Pinch freshly ground black pepper
2 cloves garlic, finely chopped
2 teaspoons fresh rosemary leaves, chopped, or 1 teaspoon dried
    rosemary, crushed
Olive oil cooking spray
Capers (optional)
Fresh rosemary sprigs (optional)

Cut the fish into 4 equal-size portions. Combine the olive oil, lemon juice, salt, pepper, garlic, and fresh or dried rosemary in a bowl and brush the mixture onto the fish.

To barbecue, arrange the fish on a barbecue rack or use a wire basket sprayed with olive oil cooking spray. Cook over medium-hot coals until the fish flakes easily (allow 4–6 minutes per 1cm/½ inch of thickness). If the fish is more than 2.5cm (1 inch) thick, gently turn it halfway through cooking.

To grill, spray the rack of a grill tray with olive oil cooking spray and arrange the fish on it. Grill 10cm (4 inches) from the heat for 4–6 minutes per 1cm (½ inch) of thickness. If the fish is more than 2.5cm (1 inch) thick, gently turn it halfway through grilling.

To serve, top the fish with capers, if using, and garnish with rosemary sprigs, if using.

Nutrition at a Glance

Per serving: 231 calories, 23g protein, 1g carbohydrates, 15g fat, 3g saturated fat, 213mg sodium, 67mg cholesterol, 0g fibre

WHITE FISH IN SPRING ONION AND GINGER SAUCE

Serves 2

75ml (3 fl oz) dry sherry or vermouth
3 tablespoons low-salt soy sauce
2 teaspoons sesame oil
4 spring onions, finely chopped
1 teaspoon freshly grated ginger
1 teaspoon finely chopped garlic
2 white fish (cod, sole or whiting) fillets (about 450g/1 lb)

Preheat the oven to 200°C/400°F/Gas 6. Mix the sherry or vermouth, soy sauce, sesame oil, onions, ginger, and garlic in a small bowl. Place the fish fillets in an ovenproof casserole dish. Drizzle the marinade over the fish and bake for 12 minutes or just until the fish flakes easily.

Nutrition at a Glance

Per serving: 242 calories, 35g protein, 3g carbohydrates, 6g fat, 1g saturated fat, 1154mg sodium, 45mg cholesterol, 1g fibre

ARMAND SALAD*

(Phase I Lunch or Dinner)

Serves 6–8

I or 2 small cloves garlic
¼ teaspoon salt
½ teaspoon pepper
I teaspoon mayonnaise
50–100ml (2–4 fl oz) fresh lemon juice
I teaspoon red wine vinegar (optional)
80ml (3 fl oz) olive oil
I head romaine lettuce, outer leaves removed, washed, dried, torn
    into bite-size pieces, and chilled
I small head iceberg lettuce, outer leaves removed, washed, dried,
    torn into bite-size pieces, and chilled
30g (1 oz) chopped fresh parsley
Onion
75g (3 oz) freshly grated Parmesan cheese, plus more for sprinkling
    on top
Thin slices of green pepper for garnish (optional)

Make the dressing in a large salad bowl: Mash the garlic, salt, and pepper to
a paste. Add the mayonnaise, continuing to mash until smooth. Then mix in
the lemon juice and the vinegar, if using. Gradually add the olive oil,
whisking.

Add the romaine and iceberg lettuce, parsley, onion, and most of the
Parmesan. Toss gently. Pile the mixture into shallow salad bowls, and
sprinkle with a little more Parmesan. Garnish with green pepper, if using,
and serve.

Nutrition at a Glance

Per serving: 176 calories, 4g protein, 4g carbohydrates, 16g fat, 3g saturated
fat, 238mg sodium, 6mg cholesterol, 2g fibre

FISH KEBABS

Serves 4

2 tablespoons extra-virgin olive oil

2 tablespoons fresh lime juice

1 tablespoon Dijon mustard

450g (1 lb) fresh halibut, swordfish, salmon, or tuna steak, cut 2.5cm
  (1 inch) thick

½ large red onion, cut lengthwise into quarters

½ green pepper, cored, seeded, and cut into 4 wedges

½ red pepper, cored, seeded, and cut into 4 wedges

4 cherry tomatoes, stemmed

Combine the oil, juice, and mustard in a 20 × 20cm (8 × 8 inch) glass baking dish; stir to blend. Cut the fish into sixteen 2.5cm (1 inch) cubes; add in one layer to marinade. Cover and marinate in the refrigerator for 5–10 minutes. Turn the fish cubes to coat evenly and chill 5 minutes longer.

Preheat the grill. Drain the fish cubes, reserving the marinade. Separate the onion layers slightly. Thread the fish and vegetables onto each of four skewers, alternating fish cubes with onions, peppers, and tomatoes. Brush the kebabs lightly with the reserved marinade.

Place the skewers on a grill tray and grill 6cm (4 inches) from the heat source, about 3 minutes. Turn the kebabs and brush again with the marinade. Grill for 3–4 minutes longer or until the fish is no longer translucent and the vegetables are tender-crisp. Serve immediately on a bed of Italian-style Spaghetti Squash (page 209).

Nutrition at a Glance

Per serving: 216 calories, 25g protein, 6g carbohydrates, 10g fat, 1g saturated fat, 158mg sodium, 36mg cholesterol, 1g fibre

GRILLED MAHI MAHI

Serves 4

450g (1 lb) mahi mahi or swordfish, fresh or frozen
2 teaspoons olive oil
2 teaspoons lemon juice
¼ teaspoon salt
Fresh ground pepper to taste
2 cloves garlic, minced
Capers (optional)

Cut the fish into 4 serving-size portions. Brush both sides of the fish with the olive oil and lemon juice. Sprinkle with salt and pepper, then rub the garlic on the fish.

To grill, arrange the fish on a grill rack and grill over medium-hot heat for 4–6 minutes per 1cm (½ inch) of thickness, or until the fish flakes easily when tested with a fork. If the fish is more than 2.5cm (1 inch) thick, gently turn it halfway through grilling.

To serve, top the fish with capers, if using.

Nutrition at a Glance

Per serving: 120 calories, 21g protein, 1g carbohydrates, 3g fat, 1g saturated fat, 245mg sodium, 83mg cholesterol, 0g fibre

OVEN-ROASTED VEGETABLES

Serves 4

1 medium courgette, cut into bite-size pieces
1 medium summer squash, cut into bite-size pieces
1 medium red pepper, cut into bite-size pieces
1 medium yellow pepper, cut into bite-size pieces
450g (1 lb) fresh asparagus, cut into bite-size pieces
1 red onion
3 tablespoons extra-virgin olive oil
1 teaspoon salt
½ teaspoon freshly ground black pepper

Heat the oven to 230°C/450°F/Gas 8. Place the courgette, squash, peppers, asparagus, and onion in a large roasting pan and toss with the olive oil, salt, and pepper to mix and coat. Spread in a single layer. Roast for 30 minutes, stirring occasionally, until the vegetables are lightly browned and tender.

Nutrition at a Glance

Per serving: 170 calories, 5g protein, 15g carbohydrates, 11g fat, 2g saturated fat, 586mg sodium, 0mg cholesterol, 5g fibre

ROASTED AUBERGINE AND PEPPERS

Serves 4

1 aubergine, peeled, halved, and sliced
2 red peppers, cut in thick strips
1 green pepper, cut in thick strips
1 onion, sliced
75ml (3 fl oz) extra-virgin olive oil
Fresh basil (optional)

Preheat oven to 180°C/350°F/Gas 4. Place the aubergine, peppers, and onion in a non-stick baking dish. Drizzle with oil, and then bake in the oven for 20 minutes, basting regularly.

Arrange the vegetables on a serving dish and garnish with fresh basil, if using.

Nutrition at a Glance

Per serving: 193 calories, 2g protein, 16g carbohydrates, 14g fat, 2g saturated fat, 5mg sodium, 0mg cholesterol, 5g fibre

SPINACH-STUFFED MUSHROOMS

Serves 8

300g (10 oz) frozen chopped spinach
⅛ teaspoon salt
8 large mushrooms
1 tablespoon extra-virgin olive oil

In a medium saucepan, bring 110ml (4 fl oz) water to a boil. Add the spinach and salt, cover, and cook according to directions on the packet. Wash the mushrooms, remove the stems and trim off the ends, then chop the stems. Heat the olive oil in a large frying pan. Add the chopped mushroom stems. Sauté until golden, about 3 minutes. Remove from the pan. Add the mushroom caps to the frying pan and sauté for 4–5 minutes. Remove the mushroom caps to a heatproof serving dish. Drain the spinach. Stir in the sautéed chopped mushrooms. Divide the spinach mixture into the caps and place in the oven on low heat to keep warm.

Nutrition at a Glance

Per serving: 33 calories, 2g protein, 3g carbohydrates, 2g fat, 0g saturated fat, 74mg sodium, 0mg cholesterol, 2g fibre

SURPRISE SOUTH BEACH MASHED 'POTATOES'

Serves 4

450g (1 lb) cauliflower florets
25g (1 oz) healthy butter-substitute spread
30ml (1 fl oz) fat-free creamer
Pinch salt
Pinch freshly ground black pepper

Steam or microwave the cauliflower until soft. Purée in a food processor, adding the 'butter' and the creamer to taste. Season with salt and pepper.

Nutrition at a Glance

Per serving: 81 calories, 2g protein, 5g carbohydrates, 6g fat, 2g saturated fat, 82mg sodium, 4mg cholesterol, 3g fibre

STEWED TOMATOES AND ONIONS

Serves 6

Lite cooking spray
60g (2 oz) chopped green pepper
30g (1 oz) thinly sliced celery
1 small onion, chopped
1 clove garlic, finely chopped
700g (1½ lb) peeled chopped tomatoes
1 tablespoon red wine vinegar
⅛ teaspoon freshly ground black pepper

Coat a large non-stick frying pan with cooking spray. Place over medium-high heat until hot. Add the pepper, celery, onion, and garlic. Sauté for 5 minutes or until the vegetables are tender. Add the tomatoes and the remaining ingredients. Bring to a boil. Cover, reduce heat, and let simmer for 15 minutes, stirring occasionally.

Nutrition at a Glance

Per serving: 29 calories, 1g protein, 7g carbohydrates, 0g fat, 0g saturated fat, 10mg sodium, 0mg cholesterol, 1g fibre

GRILLED TOMATOES

Serves 2

2 large ripe red tomatoes, halved horizontally
Pinch salt (optional)
Pinch freshly ground black pepper (optional)

Place the tomatoes on a grill tray, cut side facing up. Sprinkle with salt and pepper, if using. Grill for 7–10 minutes, until well browned.

Nutrition at a Glance

Per serving: 38 calories, 2g protein, 8g carbohydrates, 1g fat, 0g saturated fat, 16mg sodium, 0mg cholesterol, 2g fibre

GRILLED TOMATO WITH PESTO

Serves 6

3 fresh tomatoes
2 cloves garlic
30g (1 oz) chopped fresh basil leaves
2 tablespoons extra-virgin olive oil
40g (1½ oz) freshly grated Parmesan cheese
2 tablespoons pine nuts

Cut the tomatoes in half. Combine the garlic, basil, olive oil, Parmesan, and pine nuts in a blender or food processor and purée until smooth. Spoon the mixture onto the top of each tomato half. Grill the tomatoes about 7.5cm (3 inches) from the heat until lightly browned, about 3–5 minutes.

Nutrition at a Glance

Per serving: 90 calories, 3g protein, 4g carbohydrates, 7g fat, 2g saturated fat, 68mg sodium, 3mg cholesterol, 1g fibre

JOE'S MUSTARD SAUCE*

(Phase 1 condiment)

Serves 14

1 tablespoon + ½ teaspoon Colman's dry mustard, or more to taste
225g (8 oz) mayonnaise
2 teaspoons Worcestershire sauce
1 teaspoon steak sauce e.g. HP Sauce
1 tablespoon double cream
1 tablespoon milk
Salt

Place the mustard in a mixing bowl or the bowl of an electric mixer. Add the mayonnaise and beat for 1 minute. Add the Worcestershire sauce, steak sauce, cream, milk, and a pinch of salt and beat until the mixture is well-blended and creamy. If you'd like a little more mustard flavour, whisk in about ½ teaspoon more dry mustard until well blended. Chill the sauce, covered, until serving.

The stone crabs at Joe's are served cold and already cracked. They come with small metal cups of mustard sauce and melted butter. They are fabulous and great for Phase 1 if you're visiting Miami Beach!

Nutrition at a Glance

Per serving: Per tablespoon: 109 calories, 0g protein, 0g carbohydrates, 12g fat, 2g saturated fat, 87mg sodium, 6mg cholesterol, 0g fibre

EDAMAME SALAD

Serves 4

450g (1 lb) shelled edamame (green soyabeans)
50ml (2 fl oz) seasoned rice vinegar
1 tablespoon vegetable oil
¼ teaspoon salt
⅛ teaspoon freshly ground black pepper
1 bunch radishes (225g/8 oz), cut in half and thinly sliced
25g (1 oz) loosely packed chopped fresh coriander leaves

Toss the edamame, vinegar, oil, salt, pepper, radishes, and coriander together in a large bowl. Serve chilled or at room temperature.

Nutrition at a Glance

Per serving: 224 calories, 15g protein, 18g carbohydrates, 12g fat, 1g saturated fat, 479mg sodium, 0mg cholesterol, 6g fibre

ORIENTAL CABBAGE SALAD

Serves 4

½ small head green cabbage
3 spring onions, chopped
2 tablespoons dark sesame oil
2 tablespoons rice wine vinegar
2 tablespoons sesame seeds, toasted

Combine the cabbage, spring onions, oil, and vinegar. Toss well and chill until ready to serve. Add the sesame seeds and toss again before serving.

Nutrition at a Glance

Per serving: 103 calories, 2g protein, 5g carbohydrates, 9g fat, 1g saturated fat, 15mg sodium, 0mg cholesterol, 2g fibre

SNACKS

HUMMUS

Serves 5

1 tin (425g/15 oz) chick peas
2 tablespoons fresh lemon juice
110g (4 oz) tahini (sesame paste)
30g (1 oz) chopped Spanish onion
3 cloves garlic, chopped
2 teaspoons extra-virgin olive oil
2 teaspoons ground cumin
1/8 teaspoon ground paprika
1/2 teaspoon salt
Chopped fresh parsley (optional)

Drain the chick peas, reserving 50–100ml (2–4 fl oz) of the liquid.

Combine the chick peas, lemon juice, tahini, onion, garlic, oil, cumin, paprika, and salt in a blender or food processor. Purée until smooth, adding the chick pea liquid if needed to thin the purée. Refrigerate for 3–4 hours before serving to blend the flavours. Garnish with parsley, if using.

Nutrition at a Glance

Per serving: 251 calories, 8g protein, 23g carbohydrates, 16g fat, 2g saturated fat, 447mg sodium, 0mg cholesterol, 5g fibre

TURKEY ROLL-UPS

Serves 2

4 slices turkey breast
4 medium round lettuce leaves
Coriander Mayonnaise (see below)
4 spring onions
4 red pepper strips

Place I slice of turkey on each lettuce leaf spread with Coriander Mayonnaise. Add I spring onion and I pepper strip. Fold into tight, cigar-like rolls.

Ham may be substituted for the turkey. Coriander Mayonnaise can be used as a dip instead of a spread.

Nutrition at a Glance

Per serving: 54 calories, 10g protein, 2g carbohydrates, 1g fat, 0g saturated fat, 604mg sodium, 17mg cholesterol, 1g fibre

CORIANDER MAYONNAISE

Serves 10

175g (6 oz) reduced-fat (light) mayonnaise
20g (¾ oz) loosely packed coriander leaves
I tablespoon fresh lime juice
I teaspoon light soy sauce
I small clove garlic

Place the mayonnaise, coriander, lime juice, soy sauce, and garlic in a blender or food processor and blend until smooth.

Nutrition at a Glance

Per serving: 36 calories, 0g protein, 3g carbohydrates, 3g fat, 1g saturated fat, 104mg sodium, 4mg cholesterol, 0g fibre

DESSERTS

LEMON ZEST RICOTTA CRÈME

Serves 1

110g (4 oz) low-fat ricotta cheese
¼ teaspoon grated lemon zest
¼ teaspoon vanilla extract
1 sachet sugar substitute

Mix together the ricotta, lemon zest, vanilla extract, and sugar substitute in a dessert bowl. Serve chilled.

Nutrition at a Glance

Per serving: 178 calories, 14g protein, 7g carbohydrates, 10g fat, 6g saturated fat, 155mg sodium, 38mg cholesterol, 0g fibre

ALMOND RICOTTA CRÈME

Serves 1

110g (4 oz) low-fat ricotta cheese
¼ teaspoon almond extract
1 sachet sugar substitute
1 teaspoon slivered toasted almonds

Mix together the ricotta, almond extract, and sugar substitute in a dessert bowl. Serve chilled and sprinkled with toasted almonds.

Nutrition at a Glance

Per serving: 192 calories, 15g protein, 8g carbohydrates, 11g fat, 6g saturated fat, 155mg sodium, 38mg cholesterol, 0g fibre

VANILLA RICOTTA CRÈME

Serves 1

110g (4 oz) low-fat ricotta cheese
¼ teaspoon vanilla extract
1 sachet sugar substitute

Mix together the ricotta, vanilla extract, and sugar substitute in a dessert bowl. Serve chilled.

Nutrition at a Glance

Per serving: 178 calories, 14g protein, 7g carbohydrates, 10g fat, 6g saturated fat, 155mg sodium, 38mg cholesterol, 0g fibre

MOCHA RICOTTA CRÈME

Serves 1

110g (4 oz) low-fat ricotta cheese
½ teaspoon unsweetened cocoa powder
¼ teaspoon vanilla extract
1 sachet sugar substitute
Dash instant espresso powder
5 mini chocolate chips

Mix together the ricotta, cocoa powder, vanilla extract, and sugar substitute in a dessert bowl. Serve chilled with a dusting of espresso powder and sprinkle with the mini chocolate chips.

Nutrition at a Glance

Per serving: 261 calories, 15g protein, 17g carbohydrates, 14g fat, 9g saturated fat, 166mg sodium, 42mg cholesterol, 0g fibre

LIME ZEST RICOTTA CRÈME

Serves 1

110g (4 oz) low-fat ricotta cheese
¼ teaspoon grated lime zest
¼ teaspoon vanilla extract
1 sachet sugar substitute

Mix together the ricotta, lime zest, vanilla extract, and sugar substitute in a dessert bowl. Serve chilled.

Nutrition at a Glance

Per serving: 178 calories, 14g protein, 7g carbohydrates, 10g fat, 6g saturated fat, 155mg sodium, 38mg cholesterol, 0g fibre

phase 2 meal plan

We recommend that after two weeks of Phase 1, you switch to this, more liberal version of the diet. Here's where you begin to gradually reintroduce certain healthy carbs – fruit, granary bread, brown rice, wholemeal pasta, sweet potatoes – into your diet. The weight loss slows a little during Phase 2, which is why some dieters stay on Phase 1 longer than the 2-week period. If you're confident you can stick to that stricter plan for another week or two, feel free. But bear in mind that the relatively limited choices on Phase 1 make it a bad choice for a long-term diet – the danger is that you'll grow bored and be tempted to fall back into your old eating habits. You should stay on Phase 2 until you hit your target weight, at which point you move on to Phase 3. But there will be times during the course of your weight-loss regime that you will fall off the wagon – maybe you'll overindulge in sweets during a vacation, or around the holidays. Maybe there will be some stressful period that will lead you to put a few pounds back on. When that happens, we suggest that you switch back to Phase 1, just until you lose what you gained and get yourself back on track. That's how we designed the South Beach Diet – the three phases allow enough flexibility to accommodate real life.

DAY ONE

Breakfast

- 150g (6 oz) fresh strawberries
- Oatmeal (100g (4 oz) old-fashioned oatmeal mixed with 225ml (8 fl oz) skimmed milk, cooked on low heat, and sprinkled with cinnamon and 1 tablespoon chopped walnuts)
- Decaffeinated coffee or decaffeinated tea with skimmed milk and sugar substitute

Mid-morning snack

- 1 hard-boiled egg

Lunch

- Mediterranean Chicken Salad (page 189)

Mid-afternoon snack

- Fresh pear with 1 wedge Laughing Cow Light Cheese

Dinner

- Spinach-stuffed Salmon Fillet (page 206)
- Vegetable Medley (page 217)
- Tossed salad (mixed leaves, cucumber, green peppers, cherry tomatoes)
- Olive oil and vinegar to taste, or 2 tablespoons low-sugar prepared dressing

Dessert

- Chocolate-dipped Strawberries (page 219)

DAY TWO

Breakfast

- Berry smoothie (225g (8 oz) fat-free fruit-flavoured yogurt, 75g (3 oz) berries, 75g (3 oz) crushed ice; blend until smooth)
- Decaffeinated coffee or decaffeinated tea with skimmed milk and sugar substitute

Mid-morning snack

- 1 hard-boiled egg

Lunch

- Lemon Couscous Chicken (page 191)
- Tomatoes and cucumber slices

Mid-afternoon snack

- 110g (4 oz) fat-free yogurt

Dinner

- Meat Loaf (page 201)
- Steamed asparagus
- Mushrooms sautéed in olive oil
- Sliced Spanish onion and tomato with drizzled olive oil

Dessert

- Slice of melon with 2 tablespoons ricotta cheese

DAY THREE

Breakfast

- 50g (2 oz) high-fibre cereal (such as Bran Flakes) with 150ml (6 fl oz) skimmed milk
- 110g (4 oz) fresh strawberries
- Decaffeinated coffee or decaffeinated tea with skimmed milk and sugar substitute

Mid-morning snack

- Small Granny Smith apple with 1 tablespoon peanut butter

Lunch

- Greek Salad (page 128)

Mid-afternoon snack

- 110g (4 oz) fat-free yogurt

Dinner

- Herb-marinated Chicken (page 197)
- Perfection Salad (page 213)
- Steamed julienned courgette and yellow squash

Dessert

- Fresh pear with ricotta cheese and walnuts

DAY FOUR

Breakfast

- ½ fresh grapefruit
- 1 slice toasted wholemeal bread topped with 30g (1 oz) sliced reduced-fat Cheddar cheese, grilled until cheese melts
- Decaffeinated coffee or decaffeinated tea with skimmed milk and sugar substitute

Mid-morning snack

- 110g (4 oz) fat-free yogurt

Lunch

- Chef's salad (at least 30g (1 oz) each turkey, roast beef, and low-fat cheese on mixed leaves)
- 2 tablespoons Balsamic Vinaigrette (page 137) or low-sugar prepared dressing

Mid-afternoon snack

- Small Granny Smith apple with 1 wedge Laughing Cow Light Cheese

Dinner

- Asian-style Chicken Packets with Vegetables (page 199)
- Oriental Cabbage Salad (page 161)

Dessert

- Almond Ricotta Crème (page 164)

DAY FIVE

Breakfast

- Berry Smoothie (225g (8 oz) fat-free fruit-flavoured yogurt, 75g (3 oz) berries, 75g (3 oz) crushed ice; blend until smooth)
- Decaffeinated coffee or decaffeinated tea with skimmed milk and sugar substitute

Mid-morning snack

- 1 hard-boiled egg

Lunch

- Open-faced roast beef sandwich (75g (3 oz) lean roast beef, lettuce, tomato, onion, mustard, 1 slice granary bread)

Mid-afternoon snack

- 110g (4 oz) fat-free yogurt

Dinner

- Stir-fry Chicken and Vegetables (page 195)
- Tossed salad (mixed leaves, cucumber, green peppers, cherry tomatoes)
- Olive oil and vinegar to taste or 2 tablespoons low-sugar prepared dressing

Dessert

- 110g (4 oz) fat-free, sugar-free dessert (e.g. Angel Delight) with 3–4 sliced strawberries

DAY SIX

Breakfast

- 150ml (6 fl oz) vegetable juice cocktail
- 1 poached egg
- 1 wholemeal muffin
- Decaffeinated coffee or decaffeinated tea with skimmed milk and sugar substitute

Mid-morning snack

- Small Granny Smith apple with 1 tablespoon peanut butter

Lunch

- 110g (4 oz) cottage cheese with ¼ cantaloupe melon, sliced
- 4 wholemeal biscuits
- Sugar-free jelly

Mid-afternoon snack

- Hummus (page 162) with raw vegetables (you may use ready-made hummus)

Dinner

- Easy Chicken in Wine Sauce (page 196)
- Italian-style Spaghetti Squash (page 209)
- Rocket, spinach, and walnut salad
- Olive oil and balsamic vinegar to taste or 2 tablespoons prepared low-sugar dressing

Dessert

- Pistachio Bark (page 220)

DAY SEVEN

Breakfast

- ¼ cantaloupe melon
- I slice toasted wholemeal bread topped with 30g (I oz) sliced reduced-fat Cheddar cheese, grilled until cheese melts
- Decaffeinated coffee or decaffeinated tea with skimmed milk and sugar substitute

Mid-morning snack

- I 10g (4 oz) fat-free yogurt

Lunch

- Tomato stuffed with tuna salad (90g (3 oz) tuna chunks in brine, I tablespoon chopped celery, I tablespoon mayonnaise), served on a bed of salad leaves

Mid-afternoon snack

- Baba Ghannouj (page 218) with raw vegetables or wrapped in a lettuce leaf

Dinner

- Marinated Rump Steak (page 144)
- Green and yellow French beans with red pepper sautéed in olive oil
- Surprise South Beach Mashed 'Potatoes' (page 158)
- Tossed salad (mixed leaves, cucumber, green peppers, cherry tomatoes)
- Olive oil and vinegar to taste or 2 tablespoons low-sugar prepared dressing

Dessert

- Sliced cantaloupe melon with lime wedge

DAY EIGHT

Breakfast

- Sunrise Parfait (page 185)
- Decaffeinated coffee or decaffeinated tea with skimmed milk and sugar substitute

Mid-morning snack

- 1 hard-boiled egg

Lunch

- Apple-Walnut Chicken Salad (page 188)

Mid-afternoon snack

- 110g (4 oz) fat-free yogurt

Dinner

- Grilled Sole in Light Cream Sauce (page 207)
- Grilled Tomato (page 159)
- Butterhead lettuce salad
- Olive oil and balsamic vinegar to taste or 2 tablespoons prepared low-sugar dressing

Dessert

- Lemon Zest Ricotta Crème (page 164)

DAY NINE

Breakfast

- Eggs Florentine (1 poached egg served on 110g (4 oz) spinach sautéed in olive oil)
- Decaffeinated coffee or decaffeinated tea with skimmed milk and sugar substitute

Mid-morning snack

- Small Granny Smith apple with 1 tablespoon peanut butter

Lunch

- Tomato-Basil Couscous Salad (page 190)

Mid-afternoon snack

- 110g (4 oz) fat-free yogurt

Dinner

- Salsa Chicken (page 198)
- Tossed salad (mixed leaves, cucumber, green peppers, cherry tomatoes)
- 2 tablespoons Balsamic Vinaigrette (page 137) or 2 tablespoons prepared low-sugar dressing

Dessert

- Chocolate Cups (page 221)

DAY TEN

Breakfast

- Oatmeal Pancake (page 185)
- Decaffeinated coffee or decaffeinated tea with skimmed milk and sugar substitute

Mid-morning snack

- Small Granny Smith apple with 1 tablespoon peanut butter

Lunch

- Chicken and Raspberry Spinach Salad (cold chicken breast left over from Day 9) (page 187)

Mid-afternoon snack

- 110g (4 oz) fat-free yogurt

Dinner

- Meat Loaf (page 201)
- Italian-style Spaghetti Squash (page 209)

Dessert

- Strawberries with sugar substitute of your choice or dollop of low-fat topping/cream

DAY ELEVEN

Breakfast

- 110g (4 oz) fresh strawberries
- 50g (2 oz) high-fibre cereal (such as Bran Flakes) with 150ml (6 fl oz) skimmed milk
- Decaffeinated coffee or decaffeinated tea with skimmed milk and sugar substitute

Mid-morning snack

- 1 hard-boiled egg

Lunch

- Turkey-tomato pitta (75g (3 oz) sliced turkey, 3 tomato slices, small handful shredded lettuce, 1 teaspoonful Dijon mustard in a wholemeal pitta)

Mid-afternoon snack

- 110g (4 oz) fat-free yogurt

Dinner

- Cod en Papillote (page 208)
- Butterhead lettuce salad
- Olive oil and balsamic vinegar to taste or 2 tablespoons prepared low-sugar dressing

Dessert

- Baked apple

DAY TWELVE

Breakfast

- ½ grapefruit
- 1 egg, any style
- 2 slice multigrain bread
- Low-sugar jam or marmalade
- Decaffeinated coffee or decaffeinated tea with skimmed milk and sugar substitute

Mid-morning snack

- 1 chunk low-fat cheese

Lunch

- Tomato Soup (page 194)
- Chopped sirloin beef patty with 1 slice tomato and 1 slice onion in ½ wholemeal pitta

Mid-afternoon snack

- Baba Ghannouj (page 218) with raw vegetables or wrapped in a lettuce leaf

Dinner

- Grilled Chicken Salad with Tzatziki Sauce (page 212)
- Grilled asparagus with drizzled olive oil
- Tossed salad (mixed leaves, cucumber, green peppers, cherry tomatoes)
- 2 tablespoons Balsamic Vinaigrette (page 137) or 2 tablespoons prepared low-sugar dressing

Dessert

- Fresh pear with ricotta cheese and walnuts

DAY THIRTEEN

Breakfast

- 110g (4 oz) blueberries
- 1 scrambled egg with tomato salsa
- Oatmeal (60g (2 oz) old-fashioned oatmeal mixed with 225ml (8 fl oz) skimmed milk, cooked on low heat, and sprinkled with cinnamon and 1 tablespoon chopped walnuts)
- Decaffeinated coffee or decaffeinated tea with skimmed milk and sugar substitute

Mid-morning snack

- 110g (4 oz) fat-free yogurt

Lunch

- Tuna salad (80g (3 oz) tuna chunks in brine, 1 tablespoon chopped celery, 1 tablespoon mayonnaise, 3 slices tomato, 3 slices onion) in a wholemeal pitta

Mid-afternoon snack

- 1 chunk low-fat cheese

Dinner

- Pan-roasted Steak and Onions (page 200)
- South Beach Salad (page 211)
- Steamed broccoli

Dessert

- Chocolate-dipped Strawberries (page 219)

DAY FOURTEEN

Breakfast

- 150ml (6 fl oz) vegetable juice cocktail
- Baked eggs in lean bacon cups
- 1 slice multigrain bread, toasted
- Decaffeinated coffee or decaffeinated tea with skimmed milk and sugar substitute

Mid-morning snack

- 110g (4 oz) fat-free yogurt

Lunch

- Portobello Pizza (page 193)

Mid-afternoon snack

- Small Granny Smith apple with 1 wedge Laughing Cow Light Cheese

Dinner

- Grilled salmon
- Couscous
- White Asparagus Salad (page 215)

Dessert

- Fresh Strawberries with Lime Zest Ricotta Crème (page 166)

Foods to Reintroduce

FRUIT
Apples
Apricots (dried)
Apricots (fresh)
Blueberries
Cantaloupe
Cherries
Grapefruit
Grapes
Kiwi
Mangoes
Oranges
Peaches
Pears
Plums
Strawberries

DAIRY
Light fruit-flavoured yogurt
Light soya milk
Nonfat or 1% milk
Plain low-fat or fat-free yogurt

STARCHES
Use sparingly
All-Bran cereal
Bran Flakes cereal
Other high-fibre cereals
Oatmeal (not instant)
Sugar-free bran muffins (no raisins)
Brown rice
Wild rice
Wholewheat pasta
Wholewheat pittas
Stone-ground pittas
Multigrain bread
Oat and bran bread
Rye bread
Wholewheat bread
Small wholegrain bagels
Green peas
Small sweet potato
Popcorn

VEGETABLES AND LEGUMES
Black-eyed beans
Pinto beans
Barley

MISCELLANEOUS
Bittersweet chocolate (sparingly)
Semisweet chocolate (sparingly)
Fat-free sugar-free pudding
Red wine

Foods to Avoid or Eat Rarely

STARCHES AND BREADS
White rice
Baked white potatoes
Instant potatoes
Dinner rolls
Refined wheat bread
Refined wheat bagel
White bread
White flour pasta
Pretzels
Rice cakes
Cornflakes
Biscuits

VEGETABLES
Beetroot
Carrots
Corn
Potatoes

FRUIT
Bananas
Fruit juice
Juice-packed canned fruit
Pineapple
Raisins
Watermelon

MISCELLANEOUS
Honey/jam
Ice-cream

phase 2 recipes

Now that you've resolved your insulin resistance and lost a dozen or so pounds, you're ready to settle into a long-term weight loss programme. Phase 2 begins gradually reintroducing carbohydrates into your diet, starting with low-glycemic index ones such as oatmeal and couscous. The recipes herein still don't recommend even good high-glycemic carbohydrates, such as sweet potatoes, whole wheat pasta or whole grain bread or rice; the diet's flexibility allows you to begin adding these unprocessed carbs into your meals as you see fit. In this phase the desserts also become more liberal, allowing, for instance, Chocolate-dipped Strawberries.

BREAKFASTS

OATMEAL PANCAKE

Serves 1

60g (2 oz) old-fashioned oatmeal
60g (2 oz) low-fat cottage cheese (or tofu)
4 egg whites
1 teaspoon vanilla extract
¼ teaspoon cinnamon
¼ teaspoon nutmeg
Lite cooking spray

Mix the oatmeal, cottage cheese, egg whites, vanilla extract, cinnamon, and nutmeg in a blender until smooth. Spray a non-stick frying pan with cooking spray. Add the batter and cook over medium heat until both sides are lightly browned.

You can top the pancake with a low-sugar syrup of your choice.

Nutrition at a Glance

Per serving: 288 calories, 28g protein, 32g carbohydrates, 4g fat, 1g saturated fat, 451mg sodium, 5mg cholesterol, 5g fibre

SUNRISE PARFAIT

Serves 2

150g (6 oz) sliced strawberries
225g (8 oz) fat-free vanilla yogurt
50g (2 oz) Bran Flakes

Layer the strawberries, yogurt, and cereal in 2 stemmed dessert glasses.

Nutrition at a Glance

Per serving: 185 calories, 8g protein, 37g carbohydrates, 1g fat, 0g saturated fat, 102mg sodium, 3mg cholesterol, 6g fibre

LUNCHES

POACHED SALMON SPINACH SALAD

Serves 4

Poached salmon left over from Poached Salmon with Cucumber-Dill
  Sauce (page 149)
2 tablespoons extra-virgin olive oil
225g (½ lb) cleaned fresh spinach
¼ teaspoon salt
⅛ teaspoon freshly ground black pepper
60g (2 oz) chopped onion
3 fresh tomatoes (about 550g/1¼ pounds), peeled, seeded and cut
  into 1cm (½ inch) pieces
1 tablespoon coarsely chopped flat-leaf parsley (optional)

Arrange the salmon on a plate. In a frying pan, heat 1 tablespoon of the oil
over medium heat. When hot, sauté the spinach for 1½ minutes. Mix in
the salt and pepper and divide the spinach among 4 plates. Heat the
remaining tablespoon of oil in the frying pan. Sauté the onion and
tomatoes over medium heat until the onion is tender, about 5–6 minutes.
Arrange the salmon on the spinach and top with the tomatoes and onion.
Garnish with parsley, if using.

Nutrition at a Glance

Per serving: 98 calories, 2g protein, 9g carbohydrates, 7g fat, 1g saturated
fat, 162mg sodium, 0mg cholesterol, 2g fibre

CHICKEN AND RASPBERRY SPINACH SALAD

Serves 4

50ml (2 fl oz) raspberry vinegar or white wine vinegar
5 tablespoons extra-virgin olive oil
1 teaspoon honey
½ teaspoon finely grated orange zest
⅛ teaspoon salt
¼ teaspoon freshly ground black pepper
4 boneless, skinless chicken breast halves (about 350g/12 oz total)
8–10 handfuls torn spinach or torn mixed leaves
75g (3 oz) fresh raspberries
1 papaya, peeled, deseeded, and sliced; or 2 medium nectarines,
   stoned and sliced; or 2 peaches, peeled, stoned, and sliced

In a screw-top jar, combine the vinegar, 4 tablespoons of the oil, honey, orange zest, salt, and pepper. Cover and shake well. Chill the dressing until serving time.

In a medium frying pan, cook the chicken in the remaining 1 tablespoon oil over medium heat for 8–10 minutes or until the chicken is tender and no longer pink, turning often to brown evenly. Remove the chicken from the frying pan. Cut into thin, bite-size strips.

In a large bowl, toss together the warm chicken strips and the spinach or mixed leaves. Shake the dressing well. Add the dressing and raspberries to the chicken mixture. Toss lightly to coat well. Divide the chicken mixture among 4 salad plates. Arrange the papaya, nectarine, or peach slices on each plate.

Nutrition at a Glance

Per serving: 320 calories, 22g protein, 16g carbohydrates, 19g fat, 3g saturated fat, 199mg sodium, 49mg cholesterol, 5g fibre

APPLE-WALNUT CHICKEN SALAD

Serves 2

150g (5 oz) precooked chicken breast, cut into 1–2cm (½–¾ inch)
　chunks
50g (2 oz) chopped celery
80g (3 oz) chopped apple
50g (2 oz) chopped walnuts
1 tablespoon raisins
75ml (3 fl oz) prepared low-sugar Italian dressing
Butterhead lettuce

In a medium bowl, gently stir together the chicken, celery, apple, walnuts, and raisins. Pour the dressing over the mixture and toss gently to coat. Serve on a bed of lettuce.

Nutrition at a Glance

Per serving: 444 calories, 27g protein, 33g carbohydrates, 25g fat, 3g saturated fat, 391mg sodium, 63mg cholesterol, 8g fibre

MEDITERRANEAN CHICKEN SALAD

Serves 6

Dressing

  110ml (4 fl oz) low-sugar prepared Italian dressing
  1 tablespoon hot Tabasco sauce
  ½ tablespoon dried mint leaves
  ¼ tablespoon mustard powder

Salad

  450g (1 lb) boneless, skinless chicken breast
  2 tablespoons extra-virgin olive oil
  350g (12 oz) prepared bulgur wheat
  150g (5 oz) chopped cucumbers
  300g (10 oz) chopped tomatoes
  115g (4 oz) finely chopped spring onions
  30g (1 oz) chopped fresh parsley
  Romaine lettuce leaves

To make the dressing: Whisk together the dressing, Tabasco, mint, and mustard powder in a small bowl. Cover and chill until ready to use.

To make the salad: In a medium frying pan, cook the chicken in the oil over medium heat for 8–10 minutes or until the chicken is tender and no longer pink, turning often to brown evenly. Remove the chicken from the frying pan. Cut into thin, bite-size cubes. Allow the chicken to cool, then refrigerate until fully chilled. Combine the chicken with the bulgur, cucumbers, tomatoes, onions, and parsley in a bowl. Serve over the lettuce with the dressing.

Nutrition at a Glance

Per serving: 220 calories, 20g protein, 18g carbohydrates, 8g fat, 1g saturated fat, 279mg sodium, 45mg cholesterol, 4g fibre

TOMATO-BASIL COUSCOUS SALAD

Serves 6

150g (5 oz) cooked couscous
1 tomato, chopped
50g (2 oz) tinned chick peas, drained and rinsed
2 spring onions, chopped
1 teaspoon extra-virgin olive oil
1 tablespoon fresh lemon juice
1 tablespoon chopped fresh basil
Lettuce

Combine the couscous, tomato, chick peas, spring onions, oil, lemon juice, and basil in a bowl, toss, and serve on a bed of lettuce.

Nutrition at a Glance

Per serving: 43 calories, 2g protein, 7g carbohydrates, 1g fat, 0g saturated fat, 0mg sodium, 0mg cholesterol, 1g fibre

LEMON COUSCOUS CHICKEN

Serves 4

280ml (10 fl oz) water
1 tablespoon extra-virgin olive oil
350g (12 oz) broccoli florets
175g (6 oz) packet couscous (e.g. Waitrose Garlic and Coriander)
350g (12 oz) chopped cooked chicken
Juice of 1 lemon (about 3 tablespoons)
¼ teaspoon lemon zest

In a large frying pan, bring the water, oil, and broccoli to a boil. Stir in the couscous, chicken, lemon juice, and lemon zest. Remove from the heat. Cover and let stand for 5 minutes. Fluff lightly with a fork. Chill well and serve cold.

Nutrition at a Glance

Per serving: 311 calories, 24g protein, 39g carbohydrates, 7g fat, 1g saturated fat, 476mg sodium, 45mg cholesterol, 3g fibre

RUMI CHOPPED SALAD WITH LEMON VINAIGRETTE*

Phase 2 Lunch or Dinner

Serves I

Salad

I beetroot
50ml (2 fl oz) sherry vinegar
I red pepper
25g (I oz) pecans
25g (I oz) kalamata olives
6 basil leaves
I shallot

Vinaigrette

50ml (2 fl oz) lemon juice
Salt
White pepper
I egg
I teaspoon Dijon mustard
80ml (3 fl oz) olive oil
80ml (3 fl oz) rapeseed oil
I head chicory, thinly sliced
I handful frisée leaves
I orange, peeled and sectioned

To make the salad: Roast the beetroot until tender and dice into small cubes. Place the excess beetroot juice in the sherry vinegar and cook to make a marinade. Strain beetroot marinade and cover the diced beetroot with it. Roast the pepper and dice. Roast the pecans and chop them, saving some whole for garnish. Cut the olives into slivers, slice the basil leaves into strips, and chop the shallot into small pieces.

To make the vinaigrette: Place the lemon juice, salt, pepper, egg, and mustard in a blender and mix. Add the olive oil and rapeseed oil slowly to create an emulsion.

Mix the chicory, frisée, orange, pepper, pecans, olives, basil, shallot, and vinaigrette. Place a mound of diced beetroot with the juice on a plate and place a mound of dressed salad on top of that. Garnish with a whole pecan.

Nutrition at a Glance

Per serving: 338 calories, 2g protein, 9g carbohydrates, 33g fat, 4g saturated fat, 120mg sodium, 35mg cholesterol, 3g fibre

PORTOBELLO PIZZA

Serves 2

1 teaspoon extra-virgin olive oil
1 clove garlic, roughly chopped
175g (6 oz) portobello mushroom caps, cleaned
Pinch salt
Pinch freshly ground black pepper
350g (12 oz) mozzarella cheese, sliced or grated
10 fresh basil leaves
2 fresh tomatoes, sliced, roasted, or grilled
Oregano leaves (optional)

Combine the oil and garlic in a small bowl and rub the mushroom caps with the mixture on all sides. Place the caps top side down to form a circle on an oiled baking sheet; season with the salt and pepper. Arrange the cheese, basil, and tomato slices alternately in a circle on top. Sprinkle with the oregano, if using. Bake at 230°C/450°F/Gas 8 until the cheese melts, about 3 minutes.

Nutrition at a Glance

Per serving: 549 calories, 36g protein, 14g carbohydrates, 40g fat, 23g saturated fat, 651mg sodium, 133mg cholesterol, 3g fibre

TOMATO SOUP

Serves 2

1 small onion, chopped
50g (2 oz) sliced mushrooms
80g (3 oz) diced ham
¼ teaspoon extra-virgin olive oil
1 clove garlic, finely chopped
⅛ teaspoon sweet paprika
Pinch allspice
425ml (15 fl oz) chicken stock
1 tin (400g/14 oz) chick peas
3 whole tomatoes, peeled

Mix the onion, mushrooms, ham, oil, garlic, paprika, and allspice in a large pan; cook for 1 minute. Add the chicken stock, chick peas, and tomatoes; cover and simmer for 15 minutes. Purée the soup in a blender.

Nutrition at a Glance

Per serving: 404 calories, 29g protein, 58g carbohydrates, 7g fat, 2g saturated fat, 1341mg sodium, 25mg cholesterol, 12g fibre

DINNERS

STIR-FRY CHICKEN AND VEGETABLES

Serves 4

3 tablespoons rapeseed oil

225g (½ lb) cooked chicken breast, cut diagonally into 3mm (⅛ inch) thick slices

300g (10 oz) mixed prepared vegetables including broccoli, green beans, red peppers, and mushrooms

2 tablespoons water

2 tablespoons soy sauce

300g (10 oz) fresh spinach

Heat a large, heavy frying pan or wok over high heat until water sizzles when dropped onto the metal. Add 1½ tablespoons of the oil and tilt the pan gently in all directions until the oil has coated the surface. When the oil is hot (not to the point of smoking), add the chicken breast slices and stir-fry for 2 minutes. Remove the chicken to a bowl. Add the remaining oil to the frying pan. When hot, add the vegetables and stir-fry for about 4 minutes, until the larger pieces are cooked through. Return the chicken to the frying pan, add the water and soy sauce, and stir-fry for an additional 2 minutes. Add the spinach. Cover the pan and steam over medium heat for 2 minutes. Using tongs, turn the spinach once, so that it heats evenly; cover and steam for an additional 2 minutes. Remove the chicken and vegetables with a slotted spoon. Spoon the liquid into small bowls and serve as a gravy or dip.

Nutrition at a Glance

Per serving: 232 calories, 23g protein, 7g carbohydrates, 13g fat, 2g saturated fat, 616mg sodium, 48mg cholesterol, 4g fibre

EASY CHICKEN IN WINE SAUCE

Serves 4

4 tablespoons extra-virgin olive oil
1 clove garlic, crushed
3 boneless, skinless chicken breast halves, cut into strips
⅛ teaspoon salt
¼ teaspoon coarsely ground black pepper
100ml (4 fl oz) dry white wine
3 medium tomatoes, sliced

In a medium frying pan, heat the oil and garlic over medium heat; sprinkle the chicken with the salt and pepper, then add to the frying pan and cook for 7–10 minutes. Add the white wine and cook for an additional 2 minutes.

Remove the chicken and place on a dish; place the tomatoes in the frying pan and sauté until tender. Place the tomatoes over the chicken and cover with the pan drippings.

Nutrition at a Glance

Per serving: 190 calories, 6g protein, 5g carbohydrates, 15g fat, 2g saturated fat, 117mg sodium, 12mg cholesterol, 1g fibre

HERB-MARINATED CHICKEN

Serves 6

6 boneless, skinless chicken breast halves
100ml (4 fl oz) white wine
2 tablespoons extra-virgin olive or rapeseed oil
1 tablespoon white vinegar
2 teaspoons dried crushed basil
1 teaspoon dried crushed oregano or tarragon
½ teaspoon onion powder
2 cloves garlic, finely chopped

Set a heavy zip-top food-storage bag in a large mixing bowl and place the chicken in the bag. Add the wine, oil, vinegar, basil, oregano or tarragon, onion powder, and garlic. Close the bag and turn to coat the chicken well. Marinate for 5–24 hours in the refrigerator, turning occasionally.

Drain the chicken, reserving the marinade. Place the chicken on an unheated rack in a grill tray. Brush with the marinade. Grill 10–12cm (4–5 inches) from the heat for about 20 minutes or until lightly browned, brushing often with the marinade. Turn the chicken and grill for 5–15 minutes more, until the chicken is tender and no longer pink.

Nutrition at a Glance

Per serving: 185 calories, 26g protein, 1g carbohydrates, 6g fat, 1g saturated fat, 75mg sodium, 66mg cholesterol, 0g fibre

SALSA CHICKEN

Serves 4

8 handfuls finely shredded iceberg lettuce
3 tablespoons chilli powder
1 teaspoon ground cumin
450g (1 lb) boneless, skinless chicken breast, cut into 2.5cm (1-inch)
    pieces
2 large egg whites
2 tablespoons extra-virgin olive oil
225g (8 oz) chunky tomato salsa
100g (4 oz) fat-free sour cream
coriander sprigs (optional)

Divide the lettuce among 4 individual plates; cover and set aside. In a large bowl, combine the chilli powder and cumin. Add the chicken; turn to coat. Then lift the chicken from the bowl, shaking off excess coating. Dip the chicken into the egg whites, then coat again with the remaining mixture. Heat the oil in a wide non-stick frying pan or wok over medium heat. When the oil is hot, add the chicken and stir-fry gently until no longer pink in the centre; cut to test (5–7 minutes). Remove from the pan; keep warm. Pour salsa into pan; reduce heat to medium and cook, stirring, until salsa is heated through and slightly thickened. Arrange chicken over lettuce; top with salsa and sour cream. Garnish with coriander sprigs, if using.

Nutrition at a Glance

Per serving: 266 calories, 32g protein, 12g carbohydrates, 10g fat, 2g saturated fat, 457mg sodium, 66mg cholesterol, 5g fibre

ASIAN-STYLE CHICKEN PACKETS WITH VEGETABLES

Serves 4

75ml (3 fl oz) dry sherry or vermouth
3 tablespoons low-salt soy sauce
2 teaspoons sesame oil
60g (2 oz) finely chopped spring onions
1 teaspoon freshly grated ginger
1 teaspoon finely chopped garlic
4 boneless, skinless chicken breast halves, cut into 1cm (½ inch) strips
1 red pepper, sliced
300g (10 oz) mange-tout
300g (10 oz) broccoli florets
1 small tin (150g/5 oz) water chestnuts

Mix the sherry or vermouth, soy sauce, oil, onions, ginger, and garlic in a small bowl. Preheat the oven to 230°C/450°F/Gas 8 or the barbecue to medium-high. Add the chicken, pepper, peas, broccoli, and water chestnuts to the sherry or vermouth mixture and toss until evenly coated. Centre ¼ of the chicken mixture on each of four 30 × 45cm (12 × 18 inch) sheets of heavy-duty aluminium foil. Bring up the foil sides; double fold the tops and ends to seal the packets. Bake for 15–18 minutes on a baking sheet in the oven or barbecue 12–14 minutes in a covered barbecue.

Nutrition at a Glance

Per serving: 244 calories, 32g protein, 16g carbohydrates, 4g fat, 1g saturated fat, 855mg sodium, 66mg cholesterol, 7g fibre

PAN-ROASTED STEAK AND ONIONS

Serves 4

1 tablespoon extra-virgin olive oil
2 tablespoons balsamic vinegar
1 tablespoon Worcestershire sauce
1 tablespoon Dijon mustard
2 cloves garlic, finely chopped
450g (1 lb) rump steak
Lite cooking spray
1 tablespoon cracked black pepper
½ teaspoon salt
225ml (8 fl oz) chicken stock (low fat if available)
1 medium onion, cut into 6mm (¼ inch) thick rings

In a large non-aluminium baking dish, combine the oil, vinegar, Worcester-shire sauce, mustard, and garlic. Add the steak; turn to coat. Cover; refrigerate, turning once in refrigerator, 30 minutes or overnight. Coat a non-stick frying pan with cooking spray; place over medium-high heat. Sprinkle the steak with pepper and salt; brown 2 minutes per side. Add half the stock; cook, turning once, 5–6 minutes per side for medium-rare. Remove the steak from the frying pan; cover loosely to keep warm. Reduce the heat to medium. To the same frying pan add the onion rings and cook until golden brown, about 4–5 minutes per side, adding the remaining stock as needed to prevent the onions from sticking. Thinly slice the steak across the grain; serve with the onions.

Nutrition at a Glance

Per serving: 239 calories, 24g protein, 7g carbohydrates, 12g fat, 4g saturated fat, 580mg sodium, 55mg cholesterol, 1g fibre

MEAT LOAF

Serves 8

1 tin (145g/5 oz) no-salt-added tomato paste
110ml (4 fl oz) dry red wine
110ml (4 fl oz) water
1 clove garlic, finely chopped
½ teaspoon dried basil leaves
¼ teaspoon dried oregano leaves
¼ teaspoon salt
450g (1 lb) minced turkey breast
110g (4 oz) rolled oats
1 egg
50g (2 oz) grated courgette

Preheat the oven to 180°C/350°F/Gas 6. Combine the tomato paste, wine, water, garlic, basil, oregano, and salt in a small saucepan. Bring to a boil; reduce heat to low. Simmer, uncovered, for 15 minutes. Set aside.

Combine the turkey, rolled oats, egg, courgette, and one-third of the tomato mixture in a large bowl. Mix well. Shape into a loaf; place into an ungreased 20 × 10cm (8 × 4 inch) loaf pan. Bake for 45 minutes. Discard any drippings. Pour half of the remaining tomato mixture over the top of the loaf. Bake for an additional 15 minutes. Place on a serving dish. Cool 10 minutes before slicing. Serve remaining tomato sauce on the side.

Nutrition at a Glance

Per serving: 188 calories, 12g protein, 12g carbohydrates, 10g fat, 3g saturated fat, 244mg sodium, 39mg cholesterol, 2g fibre

VEAL MOUTARDE*

(Phase 2 Dinner)

Serves 4

4 medium shallots, finely chopped
2 cloves garlic, finely chopped
3 teaspoons butter
2 teaspoons Dijon mustard
2 teaspoons balsamic vinegar
1 litre (2 pints) veal stock or beef bouillon
4 small vine-ripened tomatoes, peeled, deseeded, and cut into medium dice
25g (1 oz) mustard seeds
4 veal chops (300g/10 oz), excess fat removed
Salt
Freshly ground black pepper
50ml (2 fl oz) olive oil
4 sprigs fresh rosemary, fried for 10 seconds
4 cloves garlic

Sauté half of the shallots and the garlic in 1 teaspoon butter until translucent on medium heat for about 20 to 30 seconds. Add the mustard and vinegar and cook until the vinegar is almost evaporated, about 1 minute. Add the veal stock or beef bouillon and reduce by half, to about 600ml (1 pint).

Sauté the tomatoes in 2 teaspoons butter with the remaining shallots, about 1½ minutes. Add the mustard seeds. Strain the reduced veal stock through a sieve and add to the sautéed tomatoes; add salt and pepper to taste.

Season the veal chops with salt and pepper. Pan sear the veal chops with the oil for 1½ minutes on each side or until a golden brown crust appears. Place in the oven for 8–12 minutes at 180°C/350°F/Gas 6 until desired doneness. Take out of the oven and let rest for 3–4 minutes.

To serve, place each veal chop in the centre of a shallow bowl. Pour some sauce around each one and garnish with a fried rosemary sprig and a roasted garlic clove.

Nutrition at a Glance

Per serving: 340 calories, 19g protein, 13g carbohydrates, 24g fat, 5g saturated fat, 958mg sodium, 56mg cholesterol, 2g fibre

GRILLED YELLOWFIN TUNA WITH A WHITE BEAN AND OREGANO SALAD*

(Phase 2 Dinner)

Serves 4

175g (6 oz) sushi-grade yellowfin tuna
Salt
Cracked black pepper
¼ teaspoon crushed garlic
½ lemon, juice of
50ml (2 fl oz) olive oil
50ml (2 fl oz) water
1 teaspoon fresh basil, chopped
½ tablespoon dried oregano
350g (12 oz) cooked white beans (e.g. butter beans)
1 teaspoon parsley, chopped

Season the tuna with salt and pepper to taste and grill each side for 30–45 seconds. Set aside to cool. Mix the garlic, lemon juice, olive oil, water, basil, and oregano in a cold mixing bowl and let marinate for 3 hours in the refrigerator. To serve, bring the salad to room temperature. Place the salad in the middle of a shallow bowl, slice the tuna thinly, and lay it on top of the beans next to the salad. Garnish the plate with chopped parsley.

Nutrition at a Glance

Per serving: 299 calories, 18g protein, 23g carbohydrates, 15g fat, 2g saturated fat, 19mg sodium, 19mg cholesterol, 10g fibre

SHRIMP LOUIS*

(Phase 2 Lunch or Dinner; Phase I without the chick peas)

Serves 2

Prawns

  350g (¾ lb) baby or medium-sized prawns
  Salt
  I small lime, juice of
  Lettuce leaves
  100g (4 oz) tinned chick peas, drained
  I large ripe tomato, cored and sliced
  2 eggs, hard-boiled
  2 lemons, cut in half crosswise
  4 ripe black olives
  4 thin round slices green pepper

Louis Dressing

  100g (4 oz) mayonnaise
  2 tablespoons chilli sauce
  I tablespoon grated onion
  I tablespoon chopped fresh parsley
  Salt
  Pepper
  I tablespoon double cream, plus extra to reduce thickness
  ¼ teaspoon Worcestershire sauce, or to taste
  Several drops Tabasco sauce

To cook the prawns: Drop the prawns into boiling water flavoured with a little salt and lime juice and cook until just pink, usually I to 2 minutes. Drain and cool slightly; shell and devein. Place in a bowl; cover with cling film and chill.

Arrange lettuce leaves to cover two large dinner plates; at Joe's, this is made on large oval plates. Place a mound of prawns on one side and a mound of chick peas on the other. Place tomato slices in the four 'corners' of the plate. Cut the eggs lengthwise in quarters; place a quarter next to each tomato slice. Place a lemon half at the end of each plate and 2 olives at the top and bottom. Place the green pepper rings at the edges. Cover and chill if not serving immediately.

To make the Louis dressing: Combine the mayonnaise, chilli sauce, grated onion, parsley, salt, black pepper, cream, Worcestershire sauce, and Tabasco sauce; stir until blended. Chill, covered, until serving time. If too thick, stir in a little more cream. Serve the dressing separately, in a small sauceboat.

This is a good-looking plate. The Louis dressing can be used for other cold seafood too. The Louis dressing contains a large amount of mayonnaise but is not a problem if used as a dip. Don't eat it like soup!

Nutrition at a Glance

Per serving: 867 calories, 46g protein, 40g carbohydrates, 58g fat, 10g saturated fat, 1493mg sodium, 501mg cholesterol, 7g fibre

SPINACH-STUFFED SALMON FILLETS

Serves 4

4 salmon fillets (about 150g/5 oz each)
Pinch salt
Pinch freshly ground black pepper
300g (10 oz) baby spinach, coarsely chopped
2 tablespoons prepared pesto
1 tablespoon chopped dry-packed sun-dried tomatoes
1 tablespoon pine nuts
Lite cooking spray

Heat the oven to 200°C/400°F/Gas 6. Make a slit two-thirds of the way through the centre of each fillet; do not cut through the fillet. Season each fillet with salt and pepper. In a bowl, combine the spinach, pesto, tomatoes, and pine nuts. Spoon one quarter of the mixture into each slit. Arrange the fillets on a grill tray coated with cooking spray. Roast for 8–10 minutes or until the spinach mixture is heated through.

Nutrition at a Glance

Per serving: 329 calories, 32g protein, 4g carbohydrates, 20g fat, 4g saturated fat, 213mg sodium, 86mg cholesterol, 3g fibre

GRILLED SOLE IN LIGHT CREAM SAUCE

Serves 4

3 tablespoons healthy butter-substitute spread or lite cooking spray
110ml (4 fl oz) Lea & Perrins Worcestershire Sauce
165ml (6 fl oz) fat-free creamer
4 sole fillets

Place the spread or spray in a medium saucepan. Whisk in the Worcestershire sauce; bring it to a boil and reduce the sauce slightly. Stir in the creamer and keep warm. Meanwhile, preheat the grill and place the fish on an unheated rack in a grill tray. Grill 10–15cm (4–6 inches) from the heat and cook for 2–6 minutes or until it flakes easily. Remove the fish to a serving dish and spoon the sauce over the fish.

Nutrition at a Glance

Per serving: 262 calories, 27g protein, 12g carbohydrates, 11g fat, 3g saturated fat, 860mg sodium, 76mg cholesterol, 0g fibre

COD EN PAPILLOTE

Serves 2

2 cod steaks, 2.5cm (1 inch) thick (about 600g/1 lb 5 oz)
2 tablespoons lemon juice
100g (4 oz) thinly sliced mushrooms
½ small courgette, julienned
½ small red pepper, julienned
½ small onion, thinly sliced
2 tablespoons healthy butter-substitute spread
¼ teaspoon dried tarragon leaves
Pinch freshly ground black pepper

Cut out two 60cm (2-ft) lengths of baking parchment and fold each in half to make a 30cm (1-ft) square. Place 1 cod steak slightly below the middle of each square of paper. Over each steak, sprinkle half of the lemon juice, mushrooms, courgette, pepper, and onion; dot each with half the butter substitute. Fold the parchment over the fish and crimp the edges together tightly. Place the packets side by side in a microwaveable 32 × 22 × 5cm (13 × 9 × 2 inch) baking dish. Microwave on high for 6 minutes, rotating the dish a half turn after 3 minutes.

To serve, cut an X in the top of each packet with scissors and tear open. Sprinkle with tarragon and pepper.

Nutrition at a Glance

Per serving: 370 calories, 56g protein, 7g carbohydrates, 12g fat, 2g saturated fat, 260mg sodium, 130mg cholesterol, 2g fibre

ITALIAN-STYLE SPAGHETTI SQUASH

Serves 4

1kg (2 lb) spaghetti squash
2 tablespoons lemon olive oil
1 medium red onion, thinly sliced
1 courgette (225g/8 oz), cut into 1cm (½ inch) dice
4 medium tomatoes, diced
¼ teaspoon salt
¼ teaspoon coarsely ground pepper
75g (3 oz) grated Parmesan cheese (optional)
1 small lemon, sliced

Halve the spaghetti squash lengthwise; scrape out the seeds. Place the squash halves, cut sides down, and 50ml (2 fl oz) water in a glass baking dish; cover with cling film. Microwave on high for 8–10 minutes until tender; cool slightly. Meanwhile, in a large frying pan, heat 1 tablespoon of the oil; add the onion. Cook over medium-high heat for 3 minutes until the onion is translucent. Add the courgette; cook 4–5 minutes until the courgette begins to brown. Add the tomatoes, salt, and pepper. Reduce the heat; simmer gently for 10 minutes. Using a fork, scrape the squash strands into a bowl; toss with the remaining tablespoon of oil. Divide the squash among 4 pasta bowls with mounds in the centre; spoon the vegetable mixture around the squash. Drizzle with more oil, if desired, and sprinkle with Parmesan cheese, if using. Add the lemon slices.

Nutrition at a Glance

Per serving: 190 calories, 5g protein, 28g carbohydrates, 9g fat, 1g saturated fat, 199mg sodium, 0mg cholesterol, 6g fibre

BAKED TOMATOES WITH BASIL AND PARMESAN

Serves 6

6 beef tomatoes (about 700g/1 ½ lb), cut in half
3 tablespoons finely chopped fresh herbs (basil, parsley, marjoram)
50g (2 oz) dry grated breadcrumbs
75g (3 oz) grated Parmesan or Asiago cheese
2 garlic cloves, finely chopped
Pinch salt
Pinch freshly ground black pepper
3 tablespoons extra-virgin olive oil

Preheat oven to 180°C/350°F/Gas 4. Put tomatoes in a non-stick baking dish, cut side up. Combine the herbs, breadcrumbs, Parmesan or Asiago cheese, garlic, salt, pepper, and oil in a small bowl and sprinkle each tomato with an equal portion. Bake for 30 minutes or until crusty. Tomatoes will be soft yet hold a shape.

Nutrition at a Glance

Per serving: 132 calories, 4g protein, 9g carbohydrates, 9g fat, 2g saturated fat, 161mg sodium, 5mg cholesterol, 1g fibre

SOUTH BEACH SALAD

Serves 6

Vinaigrette Dressing
    3 tablespoons extra-virgin olive oil
    3 tablespoons vegetable oil
    3 tablespoons wine vinegar
    ½ teaspoon Dijon mustard
    ½ teaspoon salt
    ½ teaspoon freshly ground black pepper

Salad
    1 tin (400g/14 oz) hearts of palm, drained and sliced
    50g (2 oz) chopped green pepper
    1 tin artichoke hearts (400g/14 oz), drained and quartered
    50g (2 oz) chopped red pepper
    10 pimiento-stuffed olives, halved
    1 head round lettuce
    2 hard-boiled eggs, cut into quarters
    12 cherry tomatoes, halved

To make the vinaigrette dressing: Combine the olive oil, vegetable oil, vinegar, mustard, salt, and pepper in a screw-top jar; cover tightly and shake vigorously to mix.

To make the salad: Combine the hearts of palm, green pepper, artichoke hearts, red pepper, and olives in a bowl. Add the vinaigrette dressing and mix well; refrigerate at least 1 hour. To serve, place the salad on a bed of lettuce leaves and garnish with the egg and cherry tomatoes.

Nutrition at a Glance

Per serving: 226 calories, 7g protein, 15g carbohydrates, 17g fat, 2g saturated fat, 710mg sodium, 71mg cholesterol, 6g fibre

GRILLED CHICKEN SALAD WITH TZATZIKI SAUCE

Serves 4

Chicken

30ml (1 fl oz) extra-virgin olive oil

2 teaspoons fresh lemon juice

1 teaspoon oregano

¼ teaspoon sea salt

1 teaspoon cracked black pepper

4 boneless, skinless chicken breast halves

Tzatziki Sauce

225g (8 oz) fat-free plain yogurt

75g (3 oz) peeled, seeded, and diced cucumber

¾ teaspoon finely chopped garlic

1 tablespoon extra-virgin olive oil

1 tablespoon white vinegar

2 tablespoons chopped fresh dill

2 tablespoons chopped fresh mint

¼ teaspoon sea salt

4 handfuls shredded iceberg lettuce

1 beef tomato (150g/5 oz), chopped

To make the chicken: Combine the oil, lemon juice, oregano, salt, and pepper in a shallow dish; add the chicken. Refrigerate for 2–3 hours. Drain and discard the marinade; grill or barbecue the chicken until a thermometer inserted in the thickest portion registers 71°C/160°F and the juices run clear. Refrigerate until chilled.

To make the sauce: Combine the yogurt, cucumber, garlic, oil, vinegar, dill, mint, and salt; process in a blender or food processor until smooth. Refrigerate until chilled.

To serve, cut the chicken into matchsticks and arrange on a bed of lettuce. Place the tomato pieces on top; serve with the sauce.

Nutrition at a Glance

Per serving: 281 calories, 30g protein, 10g carbohydrates, 14g fat, 2g saturated fat, 355mg sodium, 67mg cholesterol, 1g fibre

PERFECTION SALAD

Serves 6

1 sachet unflavoured gelatine
110ml + 280ml (4 fl oz + 10 fl oz) water
50g (2 oz) sugar substitute
50ml (2 fl oz) white vinegar
½ teaspoon salt
50g (2 oz) finely shredded cabbage
75g (3 oz) chopped celery
1 pimiento, chopped

Sprinkle the gelatine on 110ml (4 fl oz) of the water in a saucepan to soften. Place over low heat and stir until the gelatine is dissolved. Remove from the heat; add the sugar substitute, the remaining water, the vinegar, and the salt. Chill to unbeaten egg-white consistency. Fold in the cabbage, celery, and pimiento. Turn into an 850ml (1½ pint) mould or individual moulds and chill until firm.

Nutrition at a Glance

Per serving: 44 calories, 2g protein, 9g carbohydrates, 0g fat, 0g saturated fat, 219mg sodium, 0mg cholesterol, 1g fibre

MACALUSO'S SALAD*

(Phase 2 Lunch)

Serves 2

2–3 romaine lettuce hearts, cut into 2.5cm (1-inch) pieces
1 red pepper, cut into 2.5cm (1-inch) pieces
1 cucumber, thinly sliced
1 medium tomato, cut into eighths
30g (2 oz) red onion, thinly sliced and cut into 2.5cm (1-inch) pieces
50ml (2 fl oz) extra-virgin olive oil, first cold-pressed
50ml (2 fl oz) very fine red wine vinegar
3 teaspoons pecorino cheese
Salt
Freshly ground black pepper
50g (2 oz) tinned chick peas

Place the lettuce hearts, pepper, cucumber, tomato, and onion in a salad bowl.

Place the olive oil, red wine vinegar, cheese, salt, and pepper in a screw-top jar and shake well. Drizzle the dressing over the salad. Add the chick peas and toss well.

Nutrition at a Glance

Per serving: 389 calories, 9g protein, 25g carbohydrates, 30g fat, 5g saturated fat, 153mg sodium, 3mg cholesterol, 9g fibre

WHITE ASPARAGUS SALAD

Serves 4

1 teaspoon chopped fresh tarragon
110g (4 oz) finely chopped, seeded tomatoes
75ml (3 fl oz) extra-virgin olive oil
1 clove garlic, finely chopped
2 tablespoons white wine vinegar
Lettuce leaves
1 jar or tin white asparagus spears (350g/12 oz), drained

In a small bowl, combine the tarragon, tomatoes, oil, garlic, and vinegar. To serve, place lettuce leaves on individual serving plates; arrange 4–6 asparagus spears on the lettuce leaves. Spoon about 3 tablespoons of the vinaigrette over the asparagus on each plate.

Nutrition at a Glance

Per serving: 193 calories, 2g protein, 5g carbohydrates, 19g fat, 3g saturated fat, 247mg sodium, 0mg cholesterol, 2g fibre

COURGETTE RIBBONS WITH DILL

4 medium courgettes (about 700g/1 ½ lb), sliced lengthwise into
   ribbons
2 tablespoons grated Parmesan cheese
2 tablespoons fresh dill, chopped
1 tablespoon extra-virgin olive oil
1 teaspoon red pepper flakes

Bring a pot of water to the boil. Add the courgettes to the boiling water
and cook for 30–60 seconds, or until just tender. Drain.

Transfer the courgettes to a serving bowl. Add the cheese, dill, oil and
red pepper flakes. Gently toss until the courgettes are coated.

Nutrition at a Glance

Per serving: 68 calories, 3g protein, 5g carbohydrates, 5g fat, 1g saturated
fat, 52mg sodium, 2mg cholesterol, 2g fibre

VEGETABLE MEDLEY

Serves 4

1 medium courgette, cut into bite-size pieces
1 medium summer squash, cut into bite-size pieces
1 medium red pepper, cut into bite-size pieces
1 medium yellow pepper, cut into bite-size pieces
450g (1 lb) fresh asparagus, cut into bite-size pieces
4 tablespoons olive oil
1 teaspoon salt
½ teaspoon fresh ground black pepper

Heat the oven to 230°C/450°F. In a large roasting pan, combine the vegetables. Add the olive oil, salt and black pepper and toss to mix and coat. Spread in a single layer. Roast for 30 minutes, stirring occasionally, until vegetables are lightly browned and tender.

Nutrition at a Glance

Per serving: 169 calories, 5g protein, 15g carbohydrates, 11g fat, 2g saturated fat, 590mg sodium, 0mg cholesterol, 5g fibre

SNACK

BABA GHANNOUJ

Serves 1

1 medium aubergine, peeled
1 clove garlic, finely chopped
1 tablespoon tahini (sesame paste)
⅛ teaspoon ground cumin
Assorted raw vegetables

Preheat the grill. Slice the aubergine crosswise into 1cm (½-inch) slices. Place the slices on a baking sheet and grill 7cm (3 inches) from the heat until soft and water beads appear on the surface. Cool and peel the slices, then purée in a blender or food processor along with the garlic, tahini, and cumin. Chill and serve with vegetables.

Nutrition at a Glance

Per serving: 213 calories, 8g protein, 32g carbohydrates, 9g fat, 1g saturated fat, 20mg sodium, 0mg cholesterol, 12g fibre

DESSERTS

CHOCOLATE-DIPPED STRAWBERRIES

Serves 2

2 squares (25g/1 oz each) dark chocolate, chopped
½ tablespoon whipping cream
Dash almond extract
8 strawberries

Combine the chocolate and the whipping cream in a glass measuring cup
or bowl. Microwave at medium power for 1 minute or until the chocolate
melts, stirring after 30 seconds. Stir in the almond extract and let cool
slightly.

Dip each strawberry into the melted chocolate, allowing the excess to
drip off. Place on a greaseproof paper-lined baking sheet. Refrigerate or
freeze for approximately 15 minutes until set.

Nutrition at a Glance

Per serving: 175 calories, 3g protein, 24g carbohydrates, 9g fat, 6g saturated
fat, 1mg sodium, 5mg cholesterol, 4g fibre

STRAWBERRIES WITH LIGHT VANILLA YOGURT

Serves 1

110g (4 oz) fat-free vanilla yogurt
110g (4 oz) chopped strawberries

Spoon the yogurt into a dessert bowl, then add the strawberries. Serve
immediately.

Nutrition at a Glance

Per serving: 85 calories, 4g protein, 16g carbohydrates, 0g fat, 0g saturated
fat, 66mg sodium, 3mg cholesterol, 2g fibre

PISTACHIO BARK

Makes 450g (1 lb); serves about 18

12 squares dark chocolate
150g (5 oz) pistachio nuts, shelled and toasted

Microwave the chocolate in a microwaveable bowl on high for 2 minutes, stirring halfway through. Stir until completely melted. Stir the nuts into the chocolate. Spoon the chocolate and nut mixture onto a greaseproof paper-lined baking sheet. Refrigerate for 1 hour until firm. Break into bite-size pieces.

Nutrition at a Glance

Per serving (25g/1 oz): 150 calories, 3g protein, 16g carbohydrates, 10g fat, 4g saturated fat, 0mg sodium, 0mg cholesterol, 2g fibre

CHOCOLATE CUPS

Serves 8

Chocolate Cups

  8 fluted paper baking cups (to fit 8cm (3 in) muffin pan cups)
  450g (1 lb) semisweet chocolate pieces
  1 tablespoon low-fat margarine

Filling

  1 packet (85g/3½ oz) sugar-free vanilla-flavoured pudding mix (e.g.
    Angel Delight)
  285ml (½ pt) skimmed milk or as directed
  Cocoa powder

To make the Chocolate Cups, first place a paper baking cup in each of the 8 cups of the muffin pan; set aside.

In a double boiler over hot, not boiling, water (or in heavy saucepan over a low heat), heat the chocolate pieces with the margarine until melted and smooth, about 5 minutes, stirring occasionally.

Starting from the top rim of each paper cup, drizzle the chocolate mixture, 1 heaped teaspoon at a time, down the side of the cup. About 3 of these teaspoonfuls will cover the entire inside of each cup. Refrigerate until chocolate is firm, about 30 minutes.

Prepare the pudding using the milk. With a rubber spatula, fold in the whipped topping. Spoon the cream filling into the chocolate cups; sprinkle with cocoa powder.

Nutrition at a Glance

Per serving: 99 calories, 2g protein, 17g carbohydrates, 3g fat, 1g saturated fat, 206mg sodium, 5mg cholesterol, 0g fibre

phase 3 meal plan

By now you should be at your ideal weight. If you've stuck with the diet, your blood chemistry should also be improved. This is the part of the plan that's meant to help you maintain the benefits you've earned by following Phases 1 and 2. This is how you'll eat for the rest of your life. Phase 3 is the most liberal stage of the diet – by now it is simply one important aspect of a healthy lifestyle rather than a weight-loss pro-gramme. At this point you should be knowledgeable enough about how the South Beach Diet works and how it interacts with your own body to enjoy all the flexibility of the plan. In other words, if you want it, and it doesn't undo all your sacrifices, you should go ahead and enjoy. There will always be times when you overindulge a little, even after years on the diet. Those are the times when you'll switch back to Phase 1 for a week or two. You'll get back to where you were, and then you'll return to Phase 3. Don't even think of it as backsliding – we designed the diet to allow normal human beings to eat the way they want. If for you, that means having a few too many desserts once in a while, great. Enjoy it.

DAY ONE

Breakfast

- ½ grapefruit
- 2 Vegetable Quiche Cups To Go (page 125)
- Oatmeal (60g/2 oz old-fashioned oatmeal mixed with 225ml (8 fl oz) skimmed milk, cooked on low heat, and sprinkled with cinnamon and 1 tablespoon chopped walnuts)
- Decaffeinated coffee or decaffeinated tea with skimmed milk and sugar substitute

Lunch

- Roast Beef Wrap (page 244)
- Fresh apple

Dinner

- Moroccan Grilled Chicken (page 245)
- Steamed asparagus
- Couscous
- Mediterranean Salad (page 261)
- Olive oil and vinegar to taste or 2 tablespoons low-sugar prepared dressing

Dessert

- Strawberries with Light Vanilla Yogurt (page 219)

DAY TWO

Breakfast

- Fresh orange, sliced
- I egg
- 2 slices lean bacon
- I slice granary bread
- Decaffeinated coffee or decaffeinated tea with skimmed milk and sugar substitute

Lunch

- South Beach Chopped Salad with Tuna (page 130)
- Sugar-free jelly

Dinner

- Stir-fry Chicken and Vegetables (page 195)
- Coleslaw with sesame oil

Dessert

- Lemon Zest Ricotta Crème (page 164)

DAY THREE

Breakfast

- ½ grapefruit
- Egg white omelette with salsa
- I slice multigrain bread
- Decaffeinated coffee or decaffeinated tea with skimmed milk and sugar substitute

Lunch

- Open-faced ham and Swiss cheese sandwich on rye bread
- I fresh apple

Dinner

- Grilled sirloin steak
- Creamed Spinach (page 257)
- Surprise South Beach Mashed 'Potatoes' (page 158)
- Fresh Mozzarella-Tomato Salad (page 258)

Dessert

- Chocolate-dipped Apricots (page 269)

DAY FOUR

Breakfast

- ½ grapefruit
- Oatmeal (100g/4 oz old-fashioned oatmeal mixed with 225ml/8 fl oz skimmed milk, cooked on low heat, and sprinkled with cinnamon and 1 tablespoon chopped walnuts)
- 1 poached egg
- 1 slice multigrain bread
- 1 tablespoon low-sugar jam or marmalade
- Decaffeinated coffee or decaffeinated tea with skimmed milk and sugar substitute

Lunch

- Tomato stuffed with chicken salad
- Fresh melon wedge
- 110g (4 oz) fat-free yogurt

Dinner

- Snapper (or Trout) Provençal (page 252)
- Steamed mange-tout
- Rice pilaf
- Tossed salad (mixed leaves, cucumber, green peppers, cherry tomatoes)
- Olive oil and vinegar to taste or 2 tablespoons low-sugar prepared dressing

Dessert

- Chocolate-stuffed Steamed Pear (page 268)

DAY FIVE

Breakfast

- ½ grapefruit
- Western Egg White Omelette (page 124)
- ½ wholemeal muffin
- Decaffeinated coffee or decaffeinated tea with skimmed milk and sugar substitute

Lunch

- Greek Salad (page 128)
- 110g (4 oz) fat-free raspberry yogurt

Dinner

- Beef, Pepper, and Mushroom Kebabs (page 251)
- Brown Rice
- Avocado and tomato salad
- Olive oil and vinegar to taste

Dessert

- Almond Ricotta Crème (page 164)

DAY SIX

Breakfast

- Fresh blueberries
- Cinnamon Surprise (page 239)
- Decaffeinated coffee or decaffeinated tea with skimmed milk and sugar substitute

Lunch

- Chicken Caesar Salad (no croutons)
- 2 tablespoons prepared Caesar dressing

Dinner

- Savoury Prawns on Wild Rice (page 255)
- Rocket salad
- 2 tablespoons Balsamic Vinaigrette (page 137) or low-sugar prepared dressing

Dessert

- Chocolate fondue (made with dark or semi-sweet chocolate) with fresh strawberries

DAY SEVEN

Breakfast

- Fresh orange, sliced
- Tomato and Herb Frittata (page 238)
- 1 slice multigrain toast
- 1 tablespoon low-sugar jam or marmalade
- Decaffeinated coffee or decaffeinated tea with skimmed milk and sugar substitute

Lunch

- Tuna, Cucumber, and Red Pepper Salad with Lemony Dill Dressing (page 243)
- Sugar-free jelly

Dinner

- Apricot-glazed Poussins (page 249)
- Couscous
- Butterhead lettuce salad
- Olive oil and balsamic vinegar to taste or 2 tablespoons prepared low-sugar dressing

Dessert

- Chocolate Sponge Cake (page 267)

DAY EIGHT

Breakfast

- 150ml (6 fl oz) vegetable juice cocktail
- 1 egg
- 2 slice lean bacon
- ½ wholemeal English muffin
- 1 teaspoonful low-sugar jam or marmalade
- Decaffeinated coffee or decaffeinated tea with skimmed milk and sugar substitute

Lunch

- Grilled chicken salad
- 2 tablespoons Balsamic Vinaigrette (page 137) or low-sugar prepared dressing

Dinner

- Grilled Rosemary Steak (page 250)
- Fresh steamed green beans
- Baked Tomatoes with Basil and Parmesan (page 210)
- Rocket and Watercress Salad (page 259)
- 2 tablespoons Balsamic Vinaigrette (page 137) or low-sugar prepared dressing

Dessert

- Fresh strawberries and blueberries in Chocolate Cups (page 221)

DAY NINE

Breakfast

- Fresh orange, sliced
- 2 Vegetable Quiche Cups To Go (page 125)
- 1 slice multigrain toast
- Decaffeinated coffee or decaffeinated tea with skimmed milk and sugar substitute

Lunch

- Couscous Salad with Spicy Yogurt Dressing (page 240)
- Fresh nectarine

Dinner

- Lemony Fish in Foil (page 253)
- Courgette Ribbons with Dill (page 216)
- Sliced tomato
- Sliced cantaloupe melon

Dessert

- Strawberries in Balsamic Vinegar (page 263)

DAY TEN

Breakfast

- ½ grapefruit
- Oatmeal Pancake (page 185)
- Decaffeinated coffee or decaffeinated tea with skimmed milk and sugar substitute

Lunch

- Open-faced roast beef sandwich (75g/3 oz lean roast beef, lettuce, tomato, onion, mustard, 1 slice granary bread)
- Small Granny Smith apple

Dinner

- Baked chicken breast
- Italian-style Spaghetti Squash (page 209)
- Tossed salad (mixed leaves, cucumber, green peppers, cherry tomatoes)
- Prepared low-sugar Italian dressing

Dessert

- Sliced nectarines and fresh blueberries with 110g (4 oz) fat-free vanilla yogurt

DAY ELEVEN

Breakfast

- Berry smoothie (225g/8 oz fat-free fruit-flavoured yogurt, 75g/3 oz berries, 75g/3 oz crushed ice; blend until smooth)
- Decaffeinated coffee or decaffeinated tea with skimmed milk and sugar substitute

Lunch

- Frisée and Pecan Salad (page 242)
- Turkey-tomato pitta (75g/3 oz sliced turkey, 3 tomato slices, handful shredded lettuce, 1 teaspoonful Dijon mustard in a wholemeal pitta)
- 110g (4 oz) fat-free lemon yogurt

Dinner

- Marinated London Broil (page 146)
- Grilled asparagus and peppers
- Herb-roasted new potatoes (page 262)
- Tossed salad (mixed leaves, cucumber, green peppers, cherry tomatoes)
- Olive oil and vinegar to taste or 2 tablespoons low-sugar prepared dressing

Dessert

- Individual Lime Cheesecakes (page 266)

DAY TWELVE

Breakfast

- ½ fresh grapefruit
- Tex-Mex eggs (2 eggs scrambled with grated Cheddar cheese and salsa)
- I slice granary bread, toasted
- Decaffeinated coffee or decaffeinated tea with skimmed milk and sugar substitute

Lunch

- Roast Beef Wrap (London broil left over from Day II) (page 244)
- Fresh nectarine

Dinner

- Grilled salmon with tomato salsa
- Grilled asparagus
- Tossed salad (mixed leaves, cucumber, green peppers, cherry tomatoes)
- Olive oil and vinegar to taste or 2 tablespoons low-sugar prepared dressing

Dessert

- Chocolate-dipped Apricots (page 269)

DAY THIRTEEN

Breakfast
- ½ grapefruit
- Light Spinach Frittata with Tomato Salsa (page 121)
- Decaffeinated coffee or decaffeinated tea with skimmed milk and sugar substitute

Lunch
- Red pepper stuffed with cottage cheese and chopped vegetables
- Sliced cantaloupe melon with blueberries

Dinner
- Tandoori Poussins (page 248)
- Frisée and Pecan Salad (page 242)
- Couscous
- Hummus (page 162) with toasted pitta bread and fresh vegetables (you may use ready-made hummus)

Dessert
- Pear poached in dry red wine

DAY FOURTEEN

Breakfast

- South Beach Blintz (1 egg beaten with 75g (3 oz) crumbled cottage cheese and sugar substitute to taste, fried in non-stick omelette pan with cooking spray)
- Decaffeinated coffee or decaffeinated tea with skimmed milk and sugar substitute

Lunch

- Chef's salad (at least 30g (1 oz) each ham, turkey, and low-fat Swiss cheese on mixed leaves)
- Olive oil and vinegar to taste or 2 tablespoons low-sugar prepared dressing
- 1 slice granary bread

Dinner

- Lime-baked Fish (page 254)
- Grilled Tomatoes (page 159)
- Steamed Brussels sprouts
- Artichoke salad (chilled cooked artichoke hearts with halved cherry tomatoes and chopped spring onions)
- 2 tablespoons Balsamic Vinaigrette (page 137) or low-sugar prepared dressing

Dessert

- Chocolate-dipped Strawberries (page 219)

chapter eighteen

phase 3 recipes

Once you've reached your goal you'll switch to these recipes, which now include foods such as multigrain bread, tortillas and brown rice. At this point you'll know which carbs you can eat without gaining weight, so you'll have already integrated them into your diet. You'll notice that by this phase we've put an end to the 2 daytime snacks — by now you shouldn't really need them any longer to keep you satisfied between meals. But this is also the phase that includes Chocolate Sponge Cake, which is a fair trade.

BREAKFASTS

TOMATO AND HERB FRITTATA

Serves 2

1 tablespoon Fry Light extra-virgin olive oil cooking spray
110g (4 oz) chopped plum tomatoes
30g (1 oz) chopped spring onions
3 basil leaves, chopped
1 tablespoon low-fat butter substitute
4 eggs, beaten

Coat an ovenproof 30cm (10-inch) frying pan with cooking spray and place over a medium heat until hot. Sauté the tomatoes, spring onions, and basil in the butter until tender. Reduce the heat to low; pour the eggs evenly into the frying pan over the mixture. Cover and cook for 5–7 minutes or until cooked on the bottom and almost set on the top. Transfer the frying pan to a grill and grill until the top is set, 2–3 minutes. Slide onto a serving dish; cut into wedges to serve.

Nutrition at a Glance

Per serving: 169 calories, 16g protein, 5g carbohydrates, 9g fat, 2g saturated fat, 278mg sodium, 1mg cholesterol, 1g fibre

CINNAMON SURPRISE

Serves 1

50g (2 oz) low-fat cottage cheese
1 slice multigrain bread
Peach cinnamon

Spread the cottage cheese onto the slice of bread. Sprinkle with the cinnamon and grill until bubbly, 2–3 minutes.

Nutrition at a Glance

Per serving: 87 calories, 9g protein, 12g carbohydrates, 1g fat, 0g saturated fat, 347mg sodium, 5mg cholesterol, 3g fibre

LUNCHES

COUSCOUS SALAD WITH SPICY YOGURT DRESSING

Serves 4

Couscous
 I tablespoon extra-virgin olive oil
 I small onion, finely chopped
 I small rib celery, finely chopped
 250g (9 oz) couscous
 400ml (14 fl oz) water

Spicy Yogurt Dressing
 3 tablespoons fresh lemon juice
 3 tablespoons fat-free plain yogurt
 I tablespoon extra-virgin olive oil
 2 teaspoons grated fresh root ginger
 I clove garlic, crushed
 I teaspoon ground cumin
 I teaspoon ground coriander
 Pinch freshly ground black pepper

Salad
 75g (3 oz) dried currants or raisins
 75g (3 oz) tinned chick peas, rinsed and drained
 75g (3 oz) chopped red pepper
 75g (3 oz) chopped green pepper
 2 tablespoons chopped fresh coriander or parsley
 2 tablespoons sliced medium spring onions
 I lemon, cut into wedges (optional)

To make the couscous: Heat the oil in a 2-litre (4-pint) saucepan over medium heat. Add the onion and celery and cook for 2–3 minutes, stirring occasionally, until the vegetables are softened. Stir in the couscous to coat with oil; cook and stir I minute until lightly toasted. Add the water; bring to a boil, stirring gently. Remove from the heat; let stand, covered, for 30 minutes until cool and the liquid is absorbed, uncovering occasionally to fluff with a fork.

To make the spicy yogurt dressing: In a large bowl, mix together the lemon juice, yogurt, oil, root ginger, garlic, cumin, coriander, and pepper. Whisk before serving.

To make the salad: Transfer the couscous to a large serving bowl; spoon the currants or raisins, chickpeas, red pepper, green pepper, coriander or parsley, and spring onions into separate mounds around the couscous. Serve with the dressing. Toss all the ingredients together at the table; garnish with the lemon wedges, if using.

Nutrition at a Glance

Per serving: 393 calories, 12g protein, 69g carbohydrates, 9g fat, 1g saturated fat, 31mg sodium, 1mg cholesterol, 8g fibre

FRISEE AND PECAN SALAD

Serves 6

3 handfuls loosely packed round lettuce
1 onion, sliced
3 handfuls loosely packed frisée
¼ teaspoon freshly ground black pepper
90g (3 oz) coarsely chopped pecans, toasted
50ml (2 fl oz) red wine vinegar
¼ teaspoon salt

Combine the lettuce, onion, frisée, and pepper in a large bowl; set aside. Add the pecans, vinegar, and salt to a frying pan and cook over low heat until thoroughly heated. Pour over the lettuce; toss gently.

Nutrition at a Glance

Per serving: 118 calories, 2g protein, 7g carbohydrates, 10g fat, 1g saturated fat, 101mg sodium, 0mg cholesterol, 3g fibre

TUNA, CUCUMBER, AND RED PEPPER SALAD WITH LEMONY DILL DRESSING

Serves 4

Lemony Dill Dressing
    50ml (2 fl oz) extra virgin olive oil
    3 tablespoons fresh lemon juice
    1–2 tablespoons chopped fresh dill
    ½ teaspoon salt
    ½ teaspoon coarsely ground black pepper

Salad
    1 medium cucumber, chopped
    1 red pepper, chopped
    2 tins (185g/6½ oz each) white tuna chunks, drained and flaked
    Romaine lettuce
    1 small lemon, peeled, seeded, and sliced

To make the lemony dill dressing: Whisk the olive oil, lemon juice, dill, salt, and black pepper together in a small bowl.

To make the salad: Combine the cucumber, pepper, and tuna in a large bowl. Set aside. Arrange the lettuce on 4 plates. Spoon the tuna mixture into the centre of each plate. Arrange the lemon around the plates. Drizzle with the dressing.

If preferred, the tuna can be substituted with fresh tomatoes.

Nutrition at a Glance

Per serving: 282 calories, 24g protein, 9g carbohydrates, 17g fat, 3g saturated fat, 640mg sodium, 39mg cholesterol, 2g fibre

ROAST BEEF WRAP

Serves 4

50g (2 oz) low-fat cream cheese
4 × 22–30cm (9–10-inch) flour tortillas
½ red onion, sliced
4 spinach leaves, washed
225g (½ lb) sliced roast beef

For each wrap, spread a small amount of the cream cheese over the surface of a tortilla. Layer the onion, spinach, and roast beef on top; fold in opposite sides of the tortilla about 4cm (1 ½ inches) and roll up from the bottom.

Nutrition at a Glance

Per serving: 300 calories, 13g protein, 42g carbohydrates, 9g fat, 3g saturated fat, 659mg sodium, 21mg cholesterol, 3g fibre

DINNERS

MOROCCAN GRILLED CHICKEN

Serves 4

50ml (2 fl oz) extra-virgin olive oil
1 teaspoon dried oregano
½ teaspoon ground allspice
½ teaspoon ground cumin
½ teaspoon ground cloves
3 cloves garlic, finely chopped
4 boneless, skinless chicken breast halves
175g (6 oz) couscous
Red Pimiento Sauce (page 246)

Combine the oil, oregano, allspice, cumin, cloves, and garlic in a large bowl. Add the chicken breasts and cover with the olive oil mixture. Cook on a preheated grill over medium heat for about 30 minutes or until the juices run clear when the chicken is pierced. Remove from the grill and keep warm.

Meanwhile, prepare the couscous according to directions on the packet. When the couscous is ready, divide it among 4 plates; thinly slice each chicken breast and fan over the couscous on each plate. Drizzle 2 tablespoons of the sauce over each chicken breast.

Nutrition at a Glance

Per serving: 429 calories, 32g protein, 37g carbohydrates, 16g fat, 2g saturated fat, 89mg sodium, 66mg cholesterol, 4g fibre

RED PIMIENTO SAUCE

Makes 8 tablespoons

100ml (4 fl oz) tinned pimientos, drained
2 tablespoons lemon juice

Combine the pimientos and lemon juice in a food processor. Process for 30–45 seconds or until the sauce is smooth. Transfer to a covered container. Serve at room temperature.

Nutrition at a Glance

Per serving: 10 calories, 0g protein, 2g carbohydrates, 0g fat, 0g saturated fat, 4mg sodium, 0mg cholesterol, 0g fibre

ROAST CHICKEN WITH SWEET GARLIC, MELTED ONIONS, AND SOUR ORANGE*

(Phase 3 Dinner)

Serves 6

1.5kg (3 lb) chicken
20 medium-sized whole garlic cloves, peeled
225ml (8 fl oz) + 3 tablespoons olive oil
1 bunch flat-leaf parsley
Zest of 1 orange
Zest of 1 lime
450g (1 lb) yuca*, peeled
2 Spanish onions, thinly sliced
450ml (1 lb) sour orange juice**
225ml (8 fl oz) rich chicken stock

Cut the chicken in half and debone. Place garlic in 50ml (2 fl oz) oil and sauté until tender. When the garlic is cool, take half of it and purée with the parsley, orange zest, lime zest, and the remaining 175ml (6 fl oz) oil. Rub the garlic mixture on to the chicken and marinate for 1 day. Cook the yuca in salted water until tender, and drain. Slowly cook the onions with a little water until soft. Reserve.

Simmer the sour orange juice over low heat until syrupy. Add the chicken stock and cook until lightly thickened. Reserve.

Bake the chicken at 180°C/350°F/Gas 4 for 45 minutes, until cooked through. Sauté the yuca in the remaining 3 tablespoons olive oil until crispy. Add the onions and the reserved garlic mixture. Place the yuca on a plate with the chicken and cover with the orange mixture.

* Yuca (also known as cassava root) is a root vegetable readily available in South Florida owing mainly to our South American and Caribbean influences. Drain the oil well and use as garnish while maintaining or losing weight. Remember, sauté, don't fry!

** Sour orange juice comes from Caribbean sour oranges known as naranjas. If unavailable, mix 100ml (4 fl oz) lemon juice with 300ml (12 fl oz) orange juice.

Nutrition at a Glance

Per serving: 630 calories, 25g protein, 50g carbohydrates, 37g fat, 8g saturated fat, 240mg sodium, 85mg cholesterol, 4g fibre

TANDOORI POUSSINS

Serves 6

3 poussins, approximately 450g (1 lb) each
1½ teaspoons chilli powder
½ teaspoon salt (optional)
Pinch freshly ground black pepper
3 tablespoons fresh lime juice
225g (8 oz) fat-free plain yogurt
3 cloves garlic, chopped
2.5cm (1 inch) fresh ginger, grated
1 small onion, coarsely chopped
1 teaspoon cumin seeds
½ teaspoon ground turmeric
1 lime, cut into wedges (optional)
Fresh coriander or parsley sprigs (optional)

Thaw the poussins if frozen. Rinse, remove the giblets (if present), and pat dry. Make several slits in the skin, then split each poussin in half along the breastbone.

Mix together 1 teaspoon of the chilli powder, salt, pepper, and lime juice. Rub the mixture all over the poultry and set aside for about 15 minutes.

In a blender, purée the yogurt, garlic, ginger, onion, cumin, turmeric, and the remaining ½ teaspoon chilli powder. Place the poultry pieces in a bowl and add the yogurt mixture. Mix well to coat all the pieces. Cover and refrigerate for at least 8 hours, turning occasionally.

Preheat the oven to 220°C/400°F/Gas 6. Place the poussins, skin side up, on a rack in a roasting pan and spoon the yogurt mixture over them. Roast until thoroughly cooked, 45–60 minutes or until the poussins are very tender. Test for doneness by pricking the skin of the thigh – the juice should run clear. Serve hot. Remove the skin before eating, and garnish with lime and coriander or parsley, if using.

Nutrition at a Glance

Per serving: 150 calories, 22g protein, 8g carbohydrates, 4g fat, 1g saturated fat, 100mg sodium, 90mg cholesterol, 1g fibre

APRICOT-GLAZED POUSSINS

Serves 4

100g (4 oz) sugar-free apricot jam
75ml (3 fl oz) fresh orange juice
50ml (2 fl oz) Fry Light extra-virgin olive oil spray
4 poussins, thawed
Pinch salt
Pinch freshly ground black pepper

Combine the jam, orange juice, and spray to make the glaze. Rinse the poussins and pat dry. Rub the cavities with salt and pepper. Place the poussins, breast side up, on a rack in a roasting pan, ensuring that they do not touch. Pour on the glaze. Roast 1 hour at 180°C/350°F/Gas 4, basting every 10 minutes or until poussins are very tender. Test for doneness by pricking the skin of the thigh; the juice should run clear. Remove the poussins from the oven and let stand for 10 minutes before serving.

Nutrition at a Glance

Per serving: 449 calories, 22g protein, 26g carbohydrates, 28g fat, 7g saturated fat, 171mg sodium, 126mg cholesterol, 1g fibre

GRILLED ROSEMARY STEAK

Serves 4

4 rump steaks
2 tablespoons fresh rosemary leaves, finely chopped
2 cloves garlic, finely chopped
1 tablespoon extra-virgin olive oil
1 teaspoon grated lemon peel
1 teaspoon coarsely ground black pepper
Fresh rosemary sprigs (optional)

Score the steaks in a diamond pattern on both sides. Mix the fresh rosemary, garlic, oil, lemon peel, and black pepper in a small bowl. Rub the mixture onto the surface of the steaks. Cover and refrigerate for 1 hour. Grill the steaks until a thermometer inserted in the centre registers 60°C/145°F for medium-rare. Cut the steaks diagonally into 1cm (½-inch) thick slices. Garnish with the rosemary sprigs, if using.

Nutrition at a Glance

Per serving: 247 calories, 21g protein, 1g carbohydrates, 17g fat, 6g saturated fat, 50mg sodium, 60mg cholesterol, 0g fibre

BEEF, PEPPER, AND MUSHROOM KEBABS

Serves 4

1 tablespoon fresh lemon juice
1 tablespoon extra-virgin olive oil
1 tablespoon water
2 teaspoons Dijon mustard
½ teaspoon chopped fresh oregano
¼ teaspoon freshly ground black pepper
450g (1 lb) sirloin steak, cut into 2.5cm (1-inch) squares
1 large red pepper, cut into 2.5cm (1-inch) pieces
12 large mushrooms
225g (½ lb) brown rice
30g (1 oz) pine nuts, toasted

In a large bowl, whisk together the lemon juice, oil, water, mustard, oregano, and black pepper. Add the steak, red pepper, and mushrooms, tossing to coat. Alternately thread the steak, red pepper, and mushrooms on each of 4 metal skewers. Set aside.

Prepare the rice according to packet directions. Keep warm. Meanwhile, place the kebabs on a barbecue over medium coals (or under the grill). Cook uncovered for 8–11 minutes or until a meat thermometer measures 60°C (145°F) for medium-rare, turning occasionally. Mix the toasted pine nuts into the rice. Serve the kebabs over the rice mixture.

Nutrition at a Glance

Per serving: 493 calories, 33g protein, 50g carbohydrates, 18g fat, 5g saturated fat, 125mg sodium, 75mg cholesterol, 4g fibre

SNAPPER PROVENÇAL

Serves 4

50ml (2 fl oz) extra-virgin olive oil
750g (1½ lb) fresh red snapper or trout fillets
75g (3 oz) kalamata olives
2½ tablespoons capers
225g (8 oz) tinned tomatoes
3 tablespoons chopped shallots
½ tablespoon fresh rosemary leaves
½ tablespoon garlic, finely chopped
75ml (3 fl oz) white wine

Preheat the oven to 230°C/450°F/Gas 8. Preheat a large sauté pan on high heat for 2–3 minutes. Pour the oil into the pan, swirling to coat. Add the fish to the sauté pan and lower the heat to medium-high. Sauté the fish for 6–10 minutes, turning once halfway through the cooking time. Remove the fish from the sauté pan when it flakes easily and gently slide the fillets onto a baking sheet. Place in the oven to keep warm. Add the olives, capers, tomatoes, and shallots to the sauté pan. Stir in the rosemary and garlic, add the wine, and sauté for 5 minutes. Remove the fillets from the oven, place on a serving dish and pour the vegetable mixture over the top.

Nutrition at a Glance

Per serving: 362 calories, 36g protein, 6g carbohydrates, 19g fat, 3g saturated fat, 543mg sodium, 63mg cholesterol, 1g fibre

LEMONY FISH IN FOIL

Serves 4

4 large white fish fillets
30g (1 oz) diced carrots
30g (1 oz) diced celery
30g (1 oz) chopped spring onion
2 tablespoons chopped fresh parsley
2 lemons, thinly sliced

Heat the oven to 180°C/350°F/Gas 4. Cut four 60cm (2-foot) lengths of foil and fold each in half to make a 30cm (1-foot) square. Place 1 fish fillet slightly below the middle of each square of foil. Sprinkle ¼ of the carrots, celery, spring onion, and parsley on each fillet. Top with lemon slices. Fold the foil over the fish and crimp the edges together slightly. Place the foil-wrapped fillets on a baking sheet and bake for 15–20 minutes or until the fish flakes easily.

Nutrition at a Glance

Per serving: 119 calories, 22g protein, 5g carbohydrates, 1g fat, 0g saturated fat, 97mg sodium, 65mg cholesterol, 1g fibre

LIME-BAKED FISH

Serves 2

225g (½ lb) fresh fish fillets
50ml (2 fl oz) fresh lime juice
1 teaspoon tarragon leaves
30g (1 oz) chopped spring onion tops

Arrange the fish fillets in a baking dish. Sprinkle with the lime juice, tarragon, and spring onion tops. Bake covered at 170°C/325°F/Gas 3 for 15–20 minutes or until the fish flakes easily.

Nutrition at a Glance

Per serving: 114 calories, 22g protein, 4g carbohydrates, 1g fat, 0g saturated fat, 80mg sodium, 65mg cholesterol, 1g fibre

SAVOURY PRAWNS ON WILD RICE

Serves 4

225g (8 oz) wild rice
450g (1 lb) uncooked prawns, peeled and deveined
2 teaspoons paprika
½ teaspoon white pepper
½ teaspoon salt
½ clove garlic, finely chopped
1 tablespoon extra-virgin olive oil
100g (4 oz) cherry tomatoes, halved
Chopped fresh parsley (optional)

Prepare the wild rice according to the packet directions. In a large bowl, combine the prawns, paprika, pepper, salt, and garlic. Mix well and set aside. Heat the oil in a frying pan until hot. Add the prawns and cook on medium heat for 30 seconds. Stir the prawns and cook for an additional 45 seconds or until opaque, stirring constantly. Remove from the heat and serve over the wild rice along with tomatoes and parsley if using.

Nutrition at a Glance

Per serving: 368 calories, 32g protein, 46g carbohydrates, 6g fat, 1g saturated fat, 467mg sodium, 172mg cholesterol, 4g fibre

ASIAN PEAR SALAD*

(Phase 3 Lunch or Dessert)

Serves 4

4 Asian pears, peeled, cored, and chopped
1 shallot, finely chopped
2½ teaspoons fresh ginger, grated
450ml (16 fl oz) water
1 vanilla pod, scored in half
3 tablespoons sherry vinegar
2 tablespoons rice vinegar
50ml (2 fl oz) soya bean oil, or olive oil if unavailable
Salt
Black pepper
225g (½ lb) baby salad leaves
1 carrot, grated (optional)

In a 1-litre (2-pint) saucepan, cook the pears with the shallot, ginger, and water over medium heat until soft. Strain and set aside to cool. Once at room temperature, purée and strain through a sieve.

Remove the seeds from the vanilla pod and mix into the purée. Add the sherry vinegar and rice vinegar and blend in an electric blender or food processor. Slowly add the oil to emulsify. Season with the salt and pepper to taste. Dice the remaining pear for garnish.

To serve, toss the baby salad leaves well with the pear mixture. Divide among 4 or 6 serving plates and garnish with grated carrot (if using) and the diced pear.

This salad is served at China Grill accompanying their famous BBQ Lamb Ribs. Its delicious combination of ingredients makes it an innovative salad in tune with the South Beach Diet.

Nutrition at a Glance

Per serving: 200 calories, 2g protein, 17g carbohydrates, 14g fat, 2g saturated fat, 20mg sodium, 0mg cholesterol, 5g fibre

CREAMED SPINACH

Serves 6

2 packets (300g/10 oz each) frozen spinach, thawed
2 small shallots, finely chopped
1 clove garlic, finely chopped
60g (3 oz) fat-free sour cream
½ teaspoon salt
¼ teaspoon coarsely ground black pepper

In a frying pan, heat the spinach over medium-high heat for about 5 minutes or until the liquid evaporates. Add the shallots and garlic; cook until tender. Reduce the heat to low and stir in the sour cream, salt, and pepper until the sour cream melts. Do not simmer.

Nutrition at a Glance

Per serving: 35 calories, 3g protein, 6g carbohydrates, 0g fat, 0g saturated fat, 282mg sodium, 0mg cholesterol, 3g fibre

FRESH MOZZARELLA-TOMATO SALAD

Serves 4

2 medium ripe tomatoes, sliced
100g (4 oz) fresh mozzarella cheese, sliced
25g (1 oz) fresh basil leaves
1 basil rosette
2 tablespoons extra-virgin olive oil
2 tablespoons balsamic vinegar
1 teaspoon cracked black pepper

Arrange the tomato, mozzarella, and basil in a rotating pattern around a basil rosette in the centre of a large serving plate. Combine the oil and vinegar and drizzle over the salad. Sprinkle with the pepper.

Nutrition at a Glance

Per serving: 163 calories, 6g protein, 5g carbohydrates, 13g fat, 5g saturated fat, 114mg sodium, 22mg cholesterol, 1g fibre

ROCKET AND WATERCRESS SALAD

Serves 4

Strawberry Chutney
150g (5 oz) strawberries, hulled and sliced
1 tablespoon balsamic vinegar
1 ½ tablespoons water
½ tablespoon cracked black pepper

Vinaigrette
1 ¼ tablespoons fresh lemon juice
1 ¼ tablespoons white wine vinegar
100ml (4 fl oz) extra-virgin olive oil
1 ¼ tablespoons cracked black pepper

Salad
2 generous handfuls rocket leaves
2 generous handfuls watercress leaves
16 strawberries, stemmed and halved
Pinch freshly ground black pepper

To make the strawberry chutney: In a saucepan over medium heat, mix together the strawberries, vinegar, water, and black pepper. Bring it to a boil and continue cooking at a low boil for 25 minutes, until slightly thickened, stirring occasionally. Cool; pour into a bowl. Cover and refrigerate.

To make the vinaigrette: In a medium bowl, mix together the lemon juice and vinegar. Whisk in the oil and pepper to blend thoroughly; cover and reserve. Whisk before serving.

To serve: In a large bowl, combine the rocket and watercress with all but 4 tablespoons of the vinaigrette. Divide the mixture among 4 plates. Dip the cut sides of 4 strawberry halves in the pepper; arrange them around the leaves with 4 more strawberry halves. Dot each plate with 1 tablespoon of the reserved vinaigrette and 2 tablespoons of the chutney.

Nutrition at a Glance

Per serving: 308 calories, 2g protein, 13g carbohydrates, 28g fat, 4g saturated fat, 22mg sodium, 0mg cholesterol, 4g fibre

MACALUSO'S-STYLE GRILLED VEAL WITH BROCCOLI RABE*

(Phase 1, 2, and 3 Dinner)

Serves 2

Grilled Veal

1 teaspoon fresh chopped basil

2 cloves finely chopped garlic

¼ teaspoon paprika

Salt

Freshly ground black pepper

3 tablespoons finest extra-virgin olive oil, first cold-pressed

2 thinly pounded veal fillets (100–150g (4 to 6 oz) each)

Broccoli Rabe

300g (10 oz) cleaned broccoli rabe (a healthy vegetable in the turnip family)

50ml (2 fl oz) extra-virgin olive oil, first cold pressed

¼ teaspoon freshly ground black pepper

¼ teaspoon salt

4 whole cloves garlic (peeled)

Pinch crushed red pepper

To cook the grilled veal: Mix the basil, garlic, paprika, salt, and pepper together with the olive oil. Place the veal in the mixture and hand stir. Place the veal on a grill and pour the remaining marinade on top. Grill over medium-high heat until done (approximately 3 minutes per side).

To make the broccoli rabe: Rinse the broccoli rabe in cold water and drain completely. Pour the oil, pepper, salt, garlic, and red pepper into a stock pot over medium heat. When the oil is heated, place the broccoli rabe in the pot and cover for 4 to 7 minutes or until tender. Place the cooked broccoli rabe on a plate and serve with the grilled veal on top.

If you can't find broccoli rabe, substitute with spinach or kale.

Nutrition at a Glance

Per serving: 357 calories, 25g protein, 9g carbohydrates, 25g fat, 4g saturated fat, 380mg sodium, 100mg cholesterol, 0g fibre

MEDITERRANEAN SALAD

Serves 4

4 handfuls prewashed romaine lettuce, torn into bite-size pieces
75g (3 oz) black olives, sliced
50g (2 oz) feta cheese, crumbled
110ml (4 fl oz) Balsamic Vinaigrette (page 137) or low-sugar prepared
    dressing

Combine the lettuce and the black olives in a large bowl. Toss well. Divide
the lettuce mixture between 4 plates, sprinkle with the cheese, and drizzle
with the vinaigrette.

Nutrition at a Glance

Per serving: 101 calories, 2g protein, 11g carbohydrates, 5g fat, 1g saturated
fat, 716mg sodium, 8mg cholesterol, 1g fibre

HERB ROASTED POTATOES

Serves 4

675g (1½ lb) small red potatoes
2 tablespoons extra-virgin olive oil
¾ teaspoon dried rosemary, crumbled
¾ teaspoon mustard powder
½ teaspoon dried sage
½ teaspoon dried thyme
¼ teaspoon pepper

Preheat the oven to 230°C/450°F or prepare the grill for direct heat. With a vegetable peeler, remove a thin strip of skin from around the centre of each potato. In a large bowl, combine the oil, rosemary, mustard, sage, thyme and pepper. Add the potatoes and toss to combine.

Cut four 12cm (5 inch) square pieces of foil. Divide the potato mixture evenly among the foil pieces. Tightly wrap the potatoes in foil. Place the packets in the oven or on the grill. Cook, turning packets once, for 30–35 minutes in the oven or for 25–30 minutes under the grill, until the potatoes are tender.

Nutrition at a Glance

Per serving: 183 calories, 5g protein, 30g carbohydrates, 7g fat, 1g saturated fat, 0mg sodium, 0mg cholesterol, 4g fibre

DESSERTS

STRAWBERRIES IN BALSAMIC VINEGAR

Serves 4

675g (1 ½ lb) strawberries, stemmed and halved
2 sachets sugar substitute
3 tablespoons balsamic vinegar
Coarsely ground black pepper
Mint sprigs (optional)

In a medium bowl, toss the strawberries, sugar substitute, and balsamic vinegar. Let stand at room temperature until ready to serve.

To serve, spoon into 4 dessert bowls; grind a little black pepper over the top. Decorate with mint sprigs, if using.

Nutrition at a Glance

Per serving: 59 calories, 1g protein, 14g carbohydrates, 1g fat, 0g saturated fat, 5mg sodium, 0mg cholesterol, 4g fibre

POACHED PEARS

Serves 4

1 packet (4-serving size) sugar-free raspberry- or strawberry-flavoured jelly
2 cups boiling water (or as directed on packet)
4 small pears, cored and peeled

In a saucepan large enough to hold all the pears, dissolve the jelly in the boiling water. Add the pears and simmer gently, covered, for 8–10 minutes. Turn them a few times so that they take on a uniform blush. Test with a cake tester or toothpick. When the pears offer no resistance when pierced, remove them with a slotted spoon. Do not overcook. Refrigerate when cool.

Pour the remaining jelly into 4 small ramekins and chill until set.

Nutrition at a Glance

Per serving: 199 calories, 11g protein, 25g carbohydrates, 1g fat, 0g saturated fat, 549mg sodium, 0mg cholesterol, 4g fibre

GINGER PEAR

Serves 8

4 medium pears, peeled, halved, and cored
50ml (2 fl oz) fresh orange juice
50g (2 oz) finely crushed gingernuts
2 tablespoons chopped walnuts
2 tablespoons melted margarine or butter

Preheat the oven to 180°C/350°F/Gas 4. Place the pear halves, cut side up, in a 30 × 19 × 5cm (12 × 7½ × 2 inch) baking dish. Drizzle the orange juice over the pears. In a small bowl, combine the gingernuts, walnuts, and the margarine or butter. Sprinkle the mixture over the pears and bake for 20–25 minutes or until the fruit is tender.

Nutrition at a Glance

Per serving: 110 calories, 1g protein, 16g carbohydrates, 5g fat, 1g saturated fat, 55mg sodium, 0mg cholesterol, 2g fibre

INDIVIDUAL LIME CHEESECAKES

Serves 12

12 round vanilla wafers
175g (6 oz) fat-free cottage cheese
225g (8 oz) Neufchâtel cheese, softened
100g (4 oz) sugar
2 eggs
1 tablespoon grated lime zest
1 tablespoon fresh lime juice
1 teaspoon vanilla extract
50g (2 oz) low-fat vanilla yogurt
2 medium kiwi fruit, peeled, sliced, and halved

Line 12 muffin tins with paper baking cases. Place 1 wafer in the bottom of each liner.

Place the cottage cheese in a blender or food processor; cover, and process until smooth. Combine cottage cheese with Neufchâtel in a medium bowl; beat at medium speed until creamy. Gradually add sugar and mix well. Add eggs, lime zest, lime juice, and vanilla extract; beat until smooth. Spoon cheese mixture evenly over vanilla wafers. Bake at 180°C/350°F/Gas 4 for 20 minutes or until cheesecakes are almost set. (Do not overbake.) Let cheesecakes cool completely on a wire rack. Remove from pans and chill thoroughly. Spread vanilla yogurt evenly over cheesecakes, and top each with 3 kiwi fruit slices.

Nutrition at a Glance

Per serving: 129 calories, 5g protein, 13g carbohydrates, 7g fat, 3g saturated fat, 161mg sodium, 51mg cholesterol, 1g fibre

CHOCOLATE SPONGE CAKE

Serves 10

7 egg whites
⅛ teaspoon cream of tartar
175g (6 oz) sugar
3 egg yolks
1 teaspoon vanilla extract
100g (4 oz) sifted flour
3 tablespoons butter, melted and cooled to lukewarm
35g (1½ oz) dark chocolate
2 tablespoons vegetable margarine

Preheat the oven to 180°C/350°F/Gas 4. Beat the egg whites with the cream of tartar in a large bowl until foamy. Beat in the sugar, 1 tablespoon at a time, until the meringue forms stiff but not dry peaks. Stir together the egg yolks and vanilla in another large bowl. Fold in one-third of the meringue. Fold in the remaining meringue until no streaks of white remain. Sprinkle the flour over the top of the mixture; fold in. Very gently fold in the melted butter; do not overfold. Turn the batter into a 25cm (10-inch) cake tin, spreading evenly. Bake for 40–45 minutes or until a wooden skewer inserted near the centre comes out clean. Run a knife around the inner and outer edges of the cake, turn out onto a rack, and cool completely with the crusty portion up.

   Melt the chocolate together with the vegetable margarine in the top of a double boiler over hot but not boiling water, stirring occasionally, until smooth. Cool slightly. Spoon the melted chocolate evenly over the top of the cake, letting the excess run down the sides.

Nutrition at a Glance

Per serving: 197 calories, 4g protein, 26g carbohydrates, 9g fat, 4g saturated fat, 76mg sodium, 73mg cholesterol, 0g fibre

CHOCOLATE-STUFFED STEAMED PEAR

Serves 2

2 ripe Bartlett or Comice pears, washed
10 dark chocolate chips

Slice the top off each pear, slightly above the widest part. Using a melon ball scoop or a small spoon, remove the core from the bottom half of the pears. Fill the hollowed pear bottoms with 5 chocolate chips each. Place the pear tops back on top of the bottoms. Stand each pear upright in an ovenproof ramekin. Place ramekins in a medium saucepan; add 2.5cm (1 inch) water to the pan. Bring the water to a simmer over medium heat. Cover the pan and let the pears steam for about 20 minutes, until translucent. Serve hot.

Nutrition at a Glance

Per serving: 179 calories, 2g protein, 35g carbohydrates, 5g fat, 2g saturated fat, 0mg sodium, 1mg cholesterol, 4g fibre

CHOCOLATE-DIPPED APRICOTS

Serves 8

50g (2 oz) dark chocolate
24 dried apricots
1 tablespoon chopped pistachios

Microwave the chocolate in a microwaveable bowl on high for 2 minutes, stirring halfway through. Stir until completely melted. Dip the apricots halfway into the chocolate. Let the excess chocolate drip off. Place the apricots onto greaseproof paper. Sprinkle the pistachios over the chocolate-covered portions of the apricots and place in the refrigerator until the chocolate is set.

Nutrition at a Glance

Per serving: 99 calories, 1g protein, 17g carbohydrates, 3g fat, 2g saturated fat, 1mg sodium, 0mg cholesterol, 2g fibre

Recipe Credits

Cherry Snapper Ceviche page 129 (Phase 1 Lunch or Dinner)
1220 at The Tides, 1220 Ocean Drive, Miami Beach. Chef: Roger Ruch

Spicy Tuna page 134 (Phase 1 Dinner)
Asian Pear Salad page 256 (Phase 3 Lunch or Dessert)
China Grill, Miami Beach. Chef: Christian Plotczyk

Florentine-style T-Bone page 143 (Phase 1 Dinner)
Grilled Yellowfin Tuna with a White Bean and Oregano Salad page 203 (Phase 2 Dinner)
Tuscan Steak, Miami Beach. Chef: Dewey Lo Sasso

Armand Salad page 152 (Phase 1 Lunch or Dinner)
Joe's Mustard Sauce page 160 (Phase 1 condiment)
Shrimp Louis page 204 (Phase 2 Lunch or Dinner; Phase 1 without the chick peas)
Joe's Stone Crab, 11 Washington Avenue, Miami Beach. Executive Chef: André Bienvenue

Veal Moutarde page 202 (Phase 2 Dinner)
Blue Door at Delano, 1685 Collins Avenue, Miami Beach. Executive Chef: Elizabeth Barlow

Rumi Chopped Salad with Lemon Vinaigrette page 192 (Phase 2 Lunch or Dinner)
Roast Chicken with Sweet Garlic, Melted Onions, and Sour Orange page 246 (Phase 3 Dinner)
Rumi Supper Club, 330 Lincoln Road, Miami Beach. Executive Chef: Scott Fredel, Co-Executive Chef: J.D. Harris

Macaluso's Salad page 214 (Phase 2 Lunch)
Macaluso's-style Grilled Veal with Broccoli Rabe page 260 (Phase 1, 2 and 3 Dinner)
Macaluso's, 1747 Alton Road, Miami Beach. Executive Chef/Owner: Michael D'Andrea

Index